So, You've Had a Stroke: Now What? A Book of Hope.

So, You've Had a Stroke: Now What? A Book of Hope.

CHRISTINE HERRICK DAVIS PhD
with contributions from Michael William Maher PhD

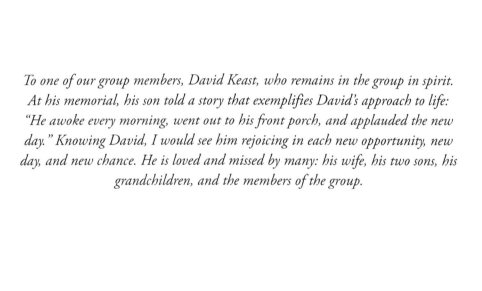

To one of our group members, David Keast, who remains in the group in spirit. At his memorial, his son told a story that exemplifies David's approach to life: "He awoke every morning, went out to his front porch, and applauded the new day." Knowing David, I would see him rejoicing in each new opportunity, new day, and new chance. He is loved and missed by many: his wife, his two sons, his grandchildren, and the members of the group.

Table of Contents

Preface · ix

One   Meet the Group · 1
Two   Incidence and Mechanism of Injury · · · · · · · · · · · · · 4

Part I   Anomia · 7
Three   The Major: The Military Approach to Stroke Recovery · · · · 9
Four   M2 also known as Michael: How My Stroke
     Got Me Out of the Dean's Office! · · · · · · · · · · · · · · · · · 16
Five   The Quarterback: I'm Too Young to Have a Stroke! · · · · · · ·47
Six   A Husband's Perspective ·55

Part II   Broca's Aphasia ·61
Seven   Barb: From Fast Track to "Slow Down and
     Smell the Roses" ·63
Eight   The Chess Master: The Doctor Had Three Strokes,
     but He's Not Out! ·73
Nine   Mike: An Engineer's Approach to Stroke Recovery · · · · · · ·83
Ten   Becky: Party On to Recovery! · · · · · · · · · · · · · · · · · · ·92

Part III   Wernicke's Aphasia ·105
Eleven   J: Closer to God ·107
Twelve   The Fly-Fisherman: Fly-Fishing through Recovery · · · · · · ·113

Part IV   Mixed Aphasia ·123

Thirteen   The Enigma: Few Words, Much Meaning · · · · · · · · · · · ·125

Fourteen   Happy-Go-Lucky: When Am I Going to Get
                  My Damn License? ·130

Fifteen   Conversations with God ·138

Part V   Living with Aphasia ·147

Sixteen   What You Should Know at Each Phase of Recovery · · · · · ·149

Seventeen   Final Thoughts on Better Outcomes · · · · · · · · · · · · · · · ·155

                  Appendix A Resources ·161

                  Appendix B Glossary ·165

                  Appendix C Additional Readings · · · · · · · · · · · · · · · · · ·173

                  Notes ·177

Preface

This book is the brainchild of Michael Maher. Michael taught in the business school at University of California, Davis and served as acting and associate dean during his twenty-eight-year tenure there. He joined the group after he had a stroke[1] that resulted in aphasia[2]—that is, it affected his ability to talk, read, and write. Although he returned to work, he was unable to get his ideas across to his colleagues as he had before. He talked haltingly at faculty meetings and kept getting interrupted. Eventually, he gave up.

In our group, he found those who were now his true colleagues. He participated enthusiastically in the group, perhaps at first to find a remedy, a cure. What he found instead was a group of individuals who together continued to work on their speech and understanding of words and, in doing so, developed a sense of peace about themselves.

Michael, in addition to being a member of the group, volunteered to teach verbs to members of the group through a computerized program being developed at the UC Davis Medical Center's aphasia clinic. Michael's love of teaching served as a way for him to feel useful, employ his strong teaching skills, and benefit the other group members. Michael recently took me aside

---

1 We use the term *stroke* as shorthand in this book for various kinds of brain injuries that may result in aphasia, such as cerebrovascular accidents (CVAs), brain tumors, and focal traumatic brain injuries.

2 Aphasia is a common sequela of stroke. It is the loss of language abilities to speak, understand language, read, and/or write. Approximately 38 percent of individuals who have a stroke also have aphasia.

and said, "You should write a book about what we are doing in the group." It was a novel idea that had never occurred to me. Throughout my career, I have written many journal articles but never a book. But I thought, "Who am I to refuse when each week I have asked all members of the group to stick their necks out and do what is most difficult for them after their strokes?" So here I am, thanks to Michael, sticking my neck out, trying something I have never done before.

I would like to acknowledge all the stroke survivors and their families who generously contributed to this book. I am particularly grateful to Maricela Cortes who helped to collect these stories and transcribe them. I am thankful to all those who read the initial stages of this book and offered suggestions and advice. These include Roxann Dehlin, Catherine Rudolph, Richard Wanlass, my husband, John, and Michael's daughter, Andrea. Finally, I want to thank Linda Boehm Vohs, who introduced me to Michael. Without that introduction, this book would not have been written.

One

Meet the Group

Thirteen of us sit around the table: a retired army major, two professors, a multilingual teacher, a famed fly-fisherman, a marketing executive, a football and basketball coach, a Hostess salesman, an internal medicine doctor, a third-grade teacher, and a banking associate. A disparate group, one might think, but we all have something in common that brings us to this room each week, where we work together for an hour and half. We are here for similar reasons, largely because we are now so similar. We all have various sorts of language problems due to suffering a stroke, brain tumor, or trauma to the brain.

The mood in the group is equal parts light and serious. One member may cry as he tells us what happened over the weekend, and at the same time, another group member laughs. There is no offense taken, just understanding and positive regard. By now we all know that with brain injury sometimes comes an inability to control one's emotions. One member will console another as we move on with the topic at hand.

This is the group, otherwise known as the Sentence Structure Group. It is not to be confused with a support group, although we do support one another. We are here to advance our expression of single words into sentences and to understand what is said more clearly and more accurately.

Groups for individuals with aphasia, like ours, exist in most major cities. They are often facilitated by speech pathologists who have experience working with aphasia. These groups vary widely in their methods and goals, but most provide a safe place for people with aphasia to feel supported as they work on improving their language skills.

I am the group facilitator, a developmental psychologist and speech pathologist, but mainly I try to stay out of the way. I bring assorted language activities to the group, newspaper articles to read, sometimes math problems, and often materials that force each of us to find a particular word or words.

This book tells the stories of the members of our group. Each person has a unique story to tell that may offer insight and encouragement to stroke survivors and their family members in a similar position. Michael and I, along with our assistant, Maricela, interviewed thirteen stroke survivors and sixteen of their family members over the course of nine months. These interviews reveal how each member survived his or her stroke, recovered, and found meaning in his or her life afterward. Their survival required a good bit of grit and a lot of grace. Although it is very serious to have a stroke, you'll see there is also ample room for humor, which some say is absolutely necessary.

These interviews address our title question: Now what? After a stroke, your specific questions may be similar to these: How will my life change? Can I go back to work after my stroke? Can I get out of my job? Am I too young to have a stroke? Who will stick with me through thick and thin? And when am I going to get my damn driver's license back?

Each chapter tells the story of one member of the group. I have inserted a prelude to each story. It is my way of describing each member and his or her particular character. Through these interviews, the stories are told by the individuals themselves. We have endeavored to keep their voices and styles intact. If we interviewed family members, their stories are included in that chapter. In this way, there are perspectives from spouses, children, and siblings.

This book is an honest look at the event of the stroke, the consequences pursuant to the stroke, the route to recovery, and the adjustments that are made day to day when stroke patients live with aphasia. It is filled with stories of the type of courage it takes to overcome a great obstacle. It is told by the members of the group who are fighting to make themselves understood—some fighting for every word.

These are not stories of miraculous recoveries. Those are the stuff of Hollywood. These stories simply illustrate the way it is for a survivor after a stroke.

A little about our group: There is an adage in neuroscience that says, "Neurons[3] that fire together wire together." This is doubly true with our Sentence Structure Group. Together we have a purpose. We work to find and express words and, as in no other adult setting, support one another in communicating.

The essential purpose of language is communication. Through the group dynamics of learning together, we strengthen our ties to one another, and this allows each of us to take a personal risk to find a word and say it aloud to others without embarrassment. We *fire together* to find the words and *wire together* in support and friendship.

---

3 Neurons are specialized cells that send nerve impulses.

Two

Incidence and Mechanism of Injury

*E*ach year approximately 795,000 people have strokes in the United States, with about three in four being first-time strokes.[4] It is the fifth-leading cause of death. The incidence of stroke is related to ethnicity and age (among other factors), with the risk of stroke increasing as we age. Women live longer, and therefore more women have strokes than men do. However, 35 percent of those who have strokes are under the age of sixty-five. High cholesterol, diabetes, hypertension, and smoking are other factors that add to stroke risk.

There are two major mechanisms of injury to the brain from a stroke: blockage of blood flow (ischemic strokes) and bleeding into the brain (hemorrhage). Blockage or interruption of blood flow in the brain results in damage through loss of oxygen to the brain cells. Eighty-seven percent of strokes are the result of ischemic causes.[5] Hemorrhage is caused by a rupture or leaking from a blood vessel in the brain and causes cell death because blood on the brain cells themselves is toxic. Approximately 13 percent of strokes are hemorrhagic.

Strokes are the leading cause of serious long-term disability.[6] Disability or deficits result when specific parts of the brain are damaged. Right-sided hemiparesis

---

4 US Centers for Disease Control and Prevention, 2017.
5 American Heart Association, 2015.
6 Ibid.

(weakness or paralysis) and aphasia are two problems associated with damage to the left part of the brain. However, not everyone who has a stroke in the left part of the brain has aphasia. It is estimated that 25–40 percent of those who have a stroke also have aphasia. Aphasia from a hemorrhagic or ischemic stroke that affects the language areas of the brain, the frontal and temporal lobes, occurs suddenly. By contrast, aphasia from a growing brain tumor is usually slower in onset. Eighty thousand new cases of aphasia are identified each year in this country, counting cases due to brain tumors and head injuries as well as stroke[7]

Orientation of MRI and CT Scans

Throughout these stories, you will see brain scans. The specific brain damage in each scan is explained. It will be helpful to refer back to this image to appreciate a normal brain scan in comparison.

The images below show the orientation of the brain when an MRI (magnetic resonance imaging) or CT (computerized tomography) scan is performed. The picture to the right is the slice of the brain taken during imaging at the level shown on the left. The resulting image on the right shows a normal brain with no abnormalities.

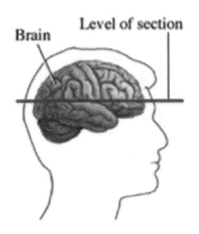 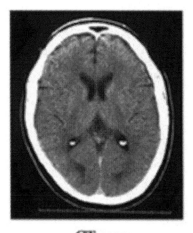

CT scan

---

7 National Stroke Association, 2008.

Part 1

ANOMIA

We are all just temporarily able bodied.

UNKNOWN

Anomia is a word-finding problem. Anomic aphasia is a type of aphasia that affects primarily expressive speech. It is characterized by obvious delays that break up the fluency of speech. During a conversation, individuals with anomia may take longer to say a word or finish a sentence. They may also use a word they didn't intend. These individuals can understand almost everything said to them unless it is lengthy or complex. In addition, they may have difficulty reading and writing. This is the mildest form of aphasia, but there is a wide variation in how it affects individuals. Some individuals may also have right-sided weakness of the arm and/or leg. This is because the damage to the brain is on the left. The left side of the brain controls the right side of the body, and therefore, if the damage spreads to the motor area of the left brain, it affects the right side of the body. Most of us process and produce language in the left temporal area of the brain, so damage here results in aphasia.

Four people in the group have this type of aphasia: the Major, Michael, Jason, and Jana.

Three

The Major: The Military Approach to Stroke Recovery

The Major is here as always, punctual and with his two reference guides. He carries *A Pocket Guide to Correct Grammar*, *A Pocket Guide to Correct English*, and an article he wants to share. His words are slowly articulated, as if he is calculating each word. His speech, as a result, has gravitas. He is perfectly groomed, baseball cap over his coifed, thick gray hair. His gaze is steady as he scans each person in the group. His style is poised and elegant, and he carries himself with an erect posture that bespeaks a major.

The Major served in Korea and Vietnam. In the military, he was an information technology (IT) expert, and he still has an interest in IT. He retired from the military in 1973. His stroke occurred when he was seventy-two.

Here is his story.

Tell us about your stroke.
My stroke was sudden, although I had some warning previously. I suffered a heart attack in 1994 and two transient ischemic attacks, or TIAs,[8] in 1996 and 2004. At the time of my first TIA, I had talked to my primary-care physician, and she sent me to [a] neurologist, but no one in the medical community thought I had a

---

8 A transient ischemic attach is a minor stroke with no residual effects.

TIA. The neurologist thought I had a balance problem, and she prescribed some exercises to restore my balance. Turns out she was wrong. On Monday, October 2004, I woke up around two o'clock in the morning, and I wondered if I had a stroke, but then I went right back to sleep. When I finally awoke that morning, I was sort of confused; I couldn't open the garage door or the front-gate latch. I had a hard time talking. My wife remembers me sitting at the dining table, eating a bowl of cereal, when I suddenly sat there with a spoon midway in my mouth. I sat there several seconds, unable to speak, when she asked if she should call the ambulance. I was unable to speak but nodded my head. The ambulance took me to Methodist Hospital in Sacramento. I was barely conscious. I had a CAT scan that same day and an MRI on the following Wednesday. [See the Major's MRI scan at end of the chapter.] I was told that I had a severe lesion in my brain, but the main thing that was affected was my speech. Later, I learned that the MRI showed that I had two TIAs previously. One of them, I believe, was while I was in Death Valley. I remember that all at once, everything was spinning. That lasted maybe for a minute. Perhaps that was a reason that I thought I had a stroke on that Monday morning in October 2004.

Was your family involved in helping you?
Both my daughters were living in the Chicago area, but they arrived at the hospital a day after my stroke. When they arrived at the hospital, I could only say a few jumbled words, could no longer read, and could no longer write my name. They took over my case. I was glad, more than glad, to have them with me. They arranged for speech therapy and physical therapy. They stayed at our house for two weeks.

At the suggestion of my speech therapist at Methodist Hospital, my daughters and granddaughter flew from Chicago to Sacramento weekly for two months, helping with appointments and speech therapy. I am more grateful to them than I can express. My wife was also supportive, but her father had a stroke, and he was bedridden at home for several years. He ultimately passed away in April 1941. I think she remembered that and thought, "It's happening again." She was devastated and was worried that she would have to take care of me. She said, "Maybe we need to find a nursing home." I reassuringly said that I didn't need that much care and that I would get better.

Did you get any therapy after your hospitalization?
After I was released from the hospital, I attended therapy. My right leg was slightly weaker than my left leg, but there was no paralysis of any sort. I had speech therapy at home for several weeks and then attended speech therapy at the outpatient clinic at Methodist Hospital from November 2004 to May 2005. At the very beginning of speech therapy, I had great difficulty finding my words. I knew what I wanted to say, but the words would not form in my brain.[9]

Sometimes, much to my family's surprise, words came out in Japanese rather than English. I [had] studied Japanese but was not fluent. For some strange reason, my sentences were sometimes a combination of English sprinkled with a few Japanese words.

At some point, my speech improvement plateaued, and my Medicare insurance was no longer going to cover the therapy expense. I was about to be cut off from speech therapy even though I was very determined to continue improving. My remarkable speech therapist at Methodist Hospital called my oldest daughter to tell her that she thought I was eager to continue and would she mind if she made some phone calls to help me find a place that I could continue this work. In August 2005, I enrolled in the Sacramento State speech-therapy program. I attribute my continued improvement to a caring speech therapist, my wife pushing me to work hard on the homework assignments I was given at therapy, and the opportunities I found at Sacramento State and UC Davis Medical Center.

As with many in our Sentence Structure Group, transportation is an issue. My neurologist said that I couldn't drive, and my wife had not driven for many years, so at first I rode Paratransit.[10] I rode Paratransit for a year but wanted an easier form of transportation where I didn't have to make a phone call to schedule the Paratransit ride. My commute took up to two hours each way.

---

9 This is a common problem in anomic aphasia.

10 Paratransit: www.paratransit.org/. Founded in 1978, Paratransit, Inc. is a local public agency organized as a nonprofit dedicated to providing transportation services to individuals with disabilities.

After two semesters at Sacramento State, I talked to my neurologist about driving, and she said if I could pass a road test, I could drive, but if I didn't pass, I would have to surrender my license then and there! Fortunately, I passed and changed my neurologist's mind.

Are there any activities you miss?

The activity I miss the most would be RVing. We had retired from the state of Texas and were living in Fairfield, California, in 1988. We were looking for a home in the Sacramento area. My wife said, "Let's buy an RV. I want to see the rest of the country before we settle down." We traveled almost twenty-six months in a pickup truck towing a fifth-wheeler. That's something I still miss. I still travel, and I even drove across country in 2013 after my wife passed away, to be with my daughters in the Chicago area. But I don't drive the fifth-wheeler anymore. Another activity I miss is reading nonfiction, like computer magazines, books on computer programming, and science books. Now I stick with fiction.

Since your stroke, how have you changed?

Since my stroke, I am mellower. I pay attention to and have more interest in my family. Of my two daughters, I am more like Barbara. We think alike, [are] both independent voters, leaning towards Democratic. Bev has my memory, and she has get-up-and-go like I do. Barbara has more outside friends. I basically have a few close friends and keep my distance from most people.

Sometimes people who have had strokes find it difficult to maintain friendships with people they knew before their speech was impaired. Skip was my close friend since 1981 and continues to be my closest friend. He has come to visit me in Chicago since I moved, and I have been able to travel by myself to visit him in Salem, Oregon, several times. He considered me his mentor. He is thirteen years younger than I am. We instantly hit it off. He understood me immediately. He is a race-car driver, which I admire. Not anything like me. Later I met SW [see chapter 12] in the group. SW and I keep in touch at least a couple times a week by e-mail. Thank God for e-mail! When I travel back to Sacramento, I really enjoy reconnecting with all the wonderful people I met in my Sentence Structure Group at UC Davis Medical Center.

How is your health now?

I am in pretty good health. My back twinges on the right side, [but it is] far better with cortisone. My doctor says, "Your blood pressure is unreal for a man your age!" My goals are to stay healthy. My prescription is to exercise a lot. I go to two group exercise classes, a private exercise class, and I walk on the treadmill at least twenty minutes a day. Otherwise, I enjoy watching movies. I watch a movie at the theater about once a week. We also have DVDs at the Reel Room at my residence. I had my first great grandchild, and I visit him once or twice a month. All my family, except my brother, who lives in Colorado Springs, lives in the North Chicago area, so I have good family connections.

I have a group of men friends, and we have dinner every Friday night. There are about twelve of us. I like to talk, general conversation. I like to stay active in my community. I go to lots of talks.

What is your advice for families?

I advise family members and spouses to be patient! A stroke victim is confused, and so are members of the family. Nobody really knows what's coming down the road.[11] And don't talk too fast, because it takes time to process any conversation. If someone says something funny, it takes me an instant to understand and respond. I can process the joke in my brain but can't get [my response] out as fast as I want to. I never felt depressed or like giving up. Life goes on; you can have a good life or a bad life, and it's up to you. I was always a go-getter; gumption I've always had. I look ahead and ask, "What's the next thing I should accomplish?"

Commentary

The Major is a good example of a very determined client. He never gives up on improving himself. I suspect he comes by this kind of discipline from his career in the military. His brain scan would predict more severe deficits in language abilities than he has. However, the Major has defied those predictions and is now considered to have primarily word-finding problems (anomic

---

11 This is a common theme you will hear throughout these stories.

aphasia[12]). The Major can make all his ideas understood but exhibits some slowness in word selection and fluency in his sentences. This points to the fact that the brain scan is useful but does not tell us everything about potential outcome.

The Major proudly asserts the following about his intelligence: "I was given an aptitude test when I was in the army that equates to an IQ test, and I scored 133 on that test." Perceived intelligence is a sore subject for the group members since they may be perceived by others as being less intelligent because of their language problems. Aphasia typically affects just language. On nonverbal cognitive tests, scores are usually within normal limits.

I have worked with the Major for over fifteen years, and it is only recently I came to learn he is a student of Zen Buddhism. I asked him in an e-mail whether he thought his interest and study of Zen Buddhism helped his recovery. This was his response:

I think the answer to your question is, probably but not consciously. I owed my college degree to the US Army, I had one year of college, in 1950/51, but I really didn't know what I wanted to do, so I took a job with a surveying crew at PG&E, in Chico, CA. I enlisted in the army in March of 1952, just ahead of the draft. I decided to stay in the army, as I was enamored with Japan.

In 1961, the army sent me to a civilian school, Orange Coast College, to study IT, then "Data Processing," for two years. I had to take a humanity class as a requirement for graduation. I decided to take "World Religions," taught by a PhD from a state college. He was well versed in the major religions, as he had traveled extensively, especially in the Far East, talking to the leaders of most of the Far East religions such as Hinduism, Jainism, and Buddhism. He was an excellent teacher, as he did not teach other religions from a Christian viewpoint. He said, "When I speak about Hinduism, I am a Hindu."

We had a lengthy test on Buddhism, including an essay question on Zen. After he graded the test, he said to me: "You either understand

---

12 Anomic aphasia is a form of aphasia that affects the efficiency word finding and sentence use.

the essence of Zen better than anyone I have ever had in this course, or you don't know anything about Zen. I don't know which." Needless to say, I got an "A" on the test. Perhaps it's a combination of my personality and my late wife's family (Japanese) that leads me toward Buddhism, especially Zen.

Today

The Major lives independently in Illinois. He drives, communicates clearly by e-mail, and participates fully in his senior-living facility. He continues to participate in an aphasia group that meets at the university. He drives from Illinois to California annually to visit his friends in the group. Since I saw him last, he appears to have gotten younger!

The Major's Brain Scan[13]

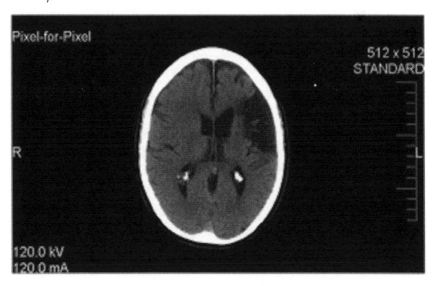

---

13 Scan orientation: The left side of the brain corresponds to the right side of the image. This image shows a left middle cerebral artery infarct, or damage involving the left frontal opercular region, left insula, and left superior temporal lobe with no midline shift of the ventricles.

Four

M2 also known as Michael: How My Stroke Got Me Out of the Dean's Office!

The former associate dean of the business school at the University of California, Davis, looks a bit like a monk, with his shaved head, on which he wears a baseball cap that says, "Stroke" with an embroidered picture of a flag on a putting green, and a T-shirt that exclaims, "Be careful or I'll put you in my book!" He exudes a quiet kindness, a professorial, understated manner. He is used to being verbally clever, and to the untrained ear, his expressive language problems would go undetected. But he elongates words as he talks as if to give himself time to self-correct before the words leave his mouth. He sometimes struggles to shape a word. Unlike most in this room, he returned to work after his stroke. He taught classes with an assistant. However, after a few years and under duress, he was urged to retire. He retired, not early really, as he is sixty-nine. However, it was not what he had hoped for. That story will be told later. Here he sits, a comfort to all of us in the group, on the ready to turn a phrase and make us all laugh.

Michael is married, a father of two girls, stepfather of two, and now grandfather of two. At the time of his stroke, he was sixty-five. He had several irons in the fire besides his deanship. He was writing a new textbook, doing research, and teaching a new class in financial accounting. Here is his story.

Tell us about the event of the stroke.

It was Wednesday, February 15, 2012. It was the day after Valentine's Day. I fell asleep about twelve midnight, and I woke up about two thirty a.m. I didn't know why I woke up, but I didn't waste time thinking about it; I immediately headed for the bathroom. But on the way to the bathroom, I thought, "Something is terribly wrong here." I found myself crashing into furniture on the way to the bathroom. I've never done that before; I thought maybe I was having inner ear problems. Same thing happened on the way back from the bathroom: I crashed into the bedroom furniture. I lay in bed for quite a while, thinking it was, perhaps, a bad dream. Soon, I would wake up from this bad dream.

I lay in bed for a while until I realized that my dizziness was not a bad dream. At three thirty a.m., I decided to test my balance again by getting up and walking to the clothes closet and to get some clothes. The same thing happened: I lost my balance going to and from the clothes closet, crashing into the bedroom furniture as I went. Everything slowed down for me. I realized, "This is serious!" I tried to talk to myself out loud and realized I couldn't. I started to panic. I was frightened, but the scary part came later.

Fortunately, my wife, Kathleen, is a sound sleeper. She has to be a sound sleeper to put up with my snoring! I didn't want to wake her up. I tried to talk again at about four o'clock in the morning. Same thing happened again: just as before, I couldn't talk! I didn't want to wake my wife up, but I wanted to ask her advice about going to the hospital. When I tried to wake her up, I discovered I still couldn't talk but could only grunt like an ape. I didn't think I had other signs of a stroke. Unbeknownst to me, awareness of them would come later.

As I shook my wife awake, she didn't panic, but she offered to take me to the hospital. She thought something was wrong, and I agreed. We got dressed to go to the hospital, and she had to tie my shoes for me. I remember riding through the sleepy town of Davis just before dawn, thinking, "It's so quiet, so peaceful" at that of time the morning. I also thought, "My wife is entitled to drive through a red light."

When we got to the emergency room at Sutter Hospital, she let me out, and I waited for her to park the car. We walked into the emergency room together. I saw a clock that read five o'clock in the morning. That's the last time I could read a clock for several days.

What happened after your admission to the ER?
After my wife filled out the paperwork, we checked into the hospital. They ran some tests, and then they declared that I had a stroke, a.k.a. brain attack. I had a blockage in my left carotid artery. I thought, OK, I was borderline high cholesterol, and my grandfather and father had strokes, so I was somewhat prepared for it. I was not panicked. I grew up on a ranch, and I saw a lot: fires broke out, houses burnt down, cows stampeding. My father was tough and taught me not to panic during a crisis; you have to be calm.

After a while the medical staff asked me when I first noticed that something was wrong. I found out later that if your stroke begins within three hours of the admittance to the hospital, for my type of ischemic stroke, the doctors could give you a drug called tPA, tissue plasminogen activator, a protein that breaks down blood clots. This can reverse the symptoms caused by a blockage in the blood flow to the brain. (I know it because it rhymes with CPA, and my wife and I are both retired CPAs.) Well, I tried to talk by grunting and groaning and tried all kinds of sign languages. The medical staff eventually gave up on my communication skills. I was trying to say, "Give me the tPA," because I knew that it would either kill me or cure me. At that point, I didn't care which. But strangely, all during this time, I was at peace with the outcome, whatever it was, to be cured, or to be killed, or even to be disabled for life. Surprisingly, I was at peace with whatever happened. I even toyed with the idea that at least now I could get out of the pressures of the associate dean's office.

The nurse's aide said it was too late. I was past the cutoff of three hours. I could tell my wife was angry. If I could, I would have lied about the onset of my stroke.

What happened after you were admitted to the hospital?
After they admitted me to the hospital, I experienced other symptoms of the stroke. I discovered I was partially blind in my right eye, I couldn't read or write, and my right hand curled up in a claw. Fortunately, there were no

problems with my lower extremities except for a loss of my balance. To this day I still lose my balance.

My wife asked me who I wanted to have at my side. I knew my colleague Shannon had cared for her parents with strokes, and I thought she would be most understanding of my situation. Through a series of gestures and sign language, I finally imparted to my wife that I wanted to have Shannon notified. I was scheduled to teach a class on Friday and Saturday, so I signaled to my wife that I also wanted to be in touch with my colleague Chelle to cover my classes.

My oldest daughter, Kai, lives in Colorado, and she flew to be with me right away. Oh my goodness, it felt great! My wife was there keeping her head when all others lose theirs. My colleague Shannon came to see me right away. I was so happy to see her. I knew she couldn't do anything special; however, she was the most knowledgeable person I could find. My second daughter, Andrea, lives in New Zealand. She was already scheduled to come for a visit in March. The doctors told us that I was out of danger of dying, so my daughter Kai told Andrea not to come until March.

My wife stayed all night with me and all the following nights that I was in the hospital. What a comfort. When I was released to the rehab center, she stayed all night with me there too. In all, there were twelve days and nights before she slept in our own bed again. My wife's presence with me in the hospital and during rehab at night was such a comfort that I'm sure it helped my recovery.

On Friday, three days after my stroke, they ran a CT scan. Then they released me from the hospital because there was a bed available at the rehab center in Roseville, California.

This was the first time I had ever ridden in an ambulance. They took me from Davis to the rehab center in Roseville, and on the way, I noticed a stop sign. I couldn't read the letters S-T-O-P. They might as well have been written in Russian. I couldn't even recognize the color red. And I certainly didn't know the shape of the stop sign; the word *octagon* wasn't in my newly altered lexicon!

What were your feelings while you were in the hospital?
I felt calm when my wife drove me to the hospital and even felt calm when they told me I had undergone a stroke. At least I could get out of the high-pressure

job I had held in the associate dean's office for so long. My feeling of serenity only lasted as long as I was in the hospital. My wife, my daughter, and the steady flow of visitors made me feel well attended to and strangely calm. I felt truly loved.

The only problem that I had in the hospital was when I was scheduled for an MRI. I am claustrophobic, so that was a big problem for me. The MRI technician was none too happy and made that known. I ended up trying to tear the machine apart, and they had to send me back for more medication. The attending nurse complained about the technician's behavior, and sometime later the hospital administration called to apologize.

What happened while you were in the rehab center?
The first weekend that I was at the rehab center, I felt like a celebrity with so many visitors. I had trouble communicating with them, but Kathleen and Kai interpreted my contorted sign language.

On Monday, we got down to my new business at hand. My physical therapist tried to get me to do as many things as possible that required coordination. First, I tried to dribble a basketball. I couldn't do that! Next, she asked me what sports I liked to play, and I said tennis. I was a pretty good tennis player before my stroke, so I picked up a tennis racket. I didn't know how to grasp the tennis racket or even what I should do with the ball. I tried to swing the racket but missed the ball.

I tried to throw darts and beanbags at a target, but I couldn't even get the mechanics down to throw anything at a target. I was so discouraged. I had intended to get over my stroke in three months, but my inability to do even the simplest of physical therapy routines left me questioning that goal.

Thinking back, [I realize] an occupational therapist helped me a lot. She had me do the mundane tasks that I would eventually need to do by myself at home, things like brushing my teeth, tying my shoes, working simple puzzles, and working on my everyday routines. This consumed all of my therapy time. The staff at the rehab center was very supportive and didn't criticize me at all.

I enjoyed the other "inmates" at the rehab center. I call them "inmates" because we didn't go outside into the real world at all. Even the prison guards were great! A couple of times, I went off the reservation by climbing stairs that I shouldn't have or practicing my balance while alone. I was pretty independent, but that didn't mean I could break out of prison yet.

An especially amusing thing happened to me that showed me I was probably trying to be too independent. After my shower on Tuesday, I decided I needed to shave. I shaved with a safety razor but without lotion or anything on my skin. I learned that in my many years of fighting fires and backpacking: I don't need any shaving cream. The combination of my ineptness and blood thinners left me bleeding all over the sink. I immediately stopped shaving, but the damage was already done. I finally stopped bloodletting in about a half an hour, just in time to go to speech therapy.

My speech therapist asked, "What happened to your chin?" I couldn't find the words to say, "I cut myself shaving." After all, I was in speech therapy, there to learn to talk. She persisted by asking, "Did you fall in the shower?" I thought about my options; probably falling while taking a shower was a lesser crime, so I nodded. She wrote that down on my chart: "Loses balance while taking a shower." Her note gave me an extension of my stay in the rehab center and an extension with my insurance. (I hope my insurance company doesn't read this part.)

My wife stayed with me during this ordeal, even eating meals with me. We found that my partial blindness did play tricks on me. For instance, I was looking all over for the cranberry juice that they served in the dining room but couldn't find it anywhere. My wife kindly said, "It's in front of you, but you can't see it, because your brain has a blockage." My wife asked me to sign my name, and it came out like this.[14] I was so proud of my signature!

Not many of us inmates were keen to venture out into the real world. But before I could be released, I had to make a trek to a shopping center. My wife and a member of the rehab therapy staff went with me. I had a lot of trouble traversing the shopping carts in the parking lot. I couldn't remember how to get from the car to the store without tripping over all of those things that kept getting in front of me.

---

14 See the writing sample at the end of the interview.

I finally made it to the store, Trader Joe's. It's a small store as stores go, but it was very confusing to me. All the stuff in the bins and on the shelves was very distracting. I felt like I was in a bazaar in India.

The therapist asked me to make a purchase, so I pulled out my billfold and looked inside. I had no idea which bills were which, so I pulled out one, just hoping it was large enough. It was large enough, and I got change back. I didn't really know what to do with my change either, but eventually I stuck it in my pocket.

I had left my safe cocoon in the hospital/rehab center for the first time in a week and a half. I felt overwhelmed, and I just wanted to go back to the calm safety of my room and my little cocoon.

On Monday, February 27, I was released, or as a medical professional says, discharged. Probably a lot of ex-cons feel like I did: what next? Or maybe it feels like a baby who is exiting the cozy, warm, comfortable womb, to go out in the cold, real world. I was eager to go home with my wife, who had been so gracious to put her life on hold for me, but I also had some trepidation.

Did you continue therapy once discharged home?
My rehab doctor admitted me to Rehab Without Walls[15] and said, "All you have to do is get well. You have no other job." I have remembered that through these following years, and it still gives me great comfort. He was a fantastic doctor. He came by to check on me on weekends and weekdays. I came to believe that he worked for me seven days a week.

I had mixed feelings about being released from the rehab center. I was glad to be home with my wife and my stepdaughter, but it was a brave new world for me. I had bouts of depression because I could not do what I had done before; I had to have help with everything. Fortunately, Rehab Without Walls came to our home seven times a week to help me. Rehab Without Walls had speech, occupational, and physical therapies. Additionally, I had a behavioral therapist, who was very helpful because I still had a lot of depression as the realities of life after the stroke set in.

---

15 Rehab Without Walls is a rehabilitation service that comes into the home to provide physical, occupational, and speech therapies.

Do you have advice for families?

My behavioral therapist turned me on to a Jodie Foster film that I had not seen before. Jodie Foster starred in *Nell,* a film about a young woman who was raised in an isolated cabin in the North Carolina mountains. Her mother was a stroke victim who died, leaving her daughter, Nell, played by Jodie Foster, to grow up without human contact and without language skills but with an abundance of emotional intelligence.

I could relate to Nell, who had the same problems with communication that I now had. In addition, I used that film to communicate to my family that I now had the same language problems as Nell. There were no problems with Nell's thinking process, but there were enduring problems with her communication. This is true for a lot of stroke patients.

We are not dumb. Talking louder is not going to make a difference, as we are not deaf. Talking slower, however, does make a difference, as it gives us a small amount of time to process what is said.

I started taking typing lessons, but I typed only the same speed as I can write, three or four words a minute. My wife told me about voice-activation software; I considered it to be a backup, but I still tried to type. Finally, after eight months I gave up trying to type. To this day I use voice-activation software. The software has a lot of problems, but I have learned to live with its problems.

Did you get adequate support from family?

My wife was my main advocate. People who have had a stroke should have one or more advocates to help negotiate with and navigate through the medical process. Kathleen stayed with me in the hospital and in the rehab center every day and night. I found that love is the best therapy of all.

My wife put her job as a lawyer on hold for one year. She dealt with my appointments, rehab, and drove me everywhere. My daughter Kai visits me frequently. She called me on the phone twice to three times a week. These were challenging phone calls. However, I think that actually her phone calls helped me continue to learn to communicate verbally more than anything else.

My daughter Andrea visited in March after my stroke. Throughout this, my extended family, consisting of my girls and a lot of cousins who came to visit me, were, and continue to be, a true godsend.

How have you continued to recover?
After I finished with Rehab Without Walls in the summer of 2012, I undertook more speech therapy with Kathy Vincent in Sacramento and with the group, also known as Sentence Structure Group, and Dr. Christine Davis.

Through a set of happy circumstances, I found the aphasia group that is administered by Dr. Davis. She was the chair of the speech-pathology department at University [of] California, Davis, while I worked there. Dr. Davis and I had two degrees of separation. We both worked at the university, but we had never met. Thankfully, we had a mutual friend who recommended me to her and her aphasia group that meets on Wednesdays.

I missed my friends at the rehab center. I felt somewhat out of place out in the real world. I thought maybe the stroke group and Dr. Davis would do me some good. I was eager to participate in the group.

The first Wednesday that I went to the stroke group, my wife accompanied me. I was very impressed with the participants and their determination: a fellow college professor, an attorney or two, a major in the army, a guy who knew six languages, a woman who was a high-level employee of the state of California, and a woman who was working for Bloomberg in San Francisco at the time she had her stroke. These participants and Dr. Davis pushed me to the limit. They were working on sentence structure, reading aloud, playing memory games, and so on. I discovered that Dr. Davis was a no-nonsense instructor. I felt that she and the members of the group could teach me a lot.

Tell us about your return to work.
I desperately wanted to go back to work at the university. My disability had earned me a year's leave through the university, so I was looking forward to getting back in the trenches in February, a year after my stroke.

Did the university support your return to work?
During the first two years after my stroke, the business school was great. But recently they have not been very supportive. I appealed to the ADA[16] department at the university level and at the business school level. At the university level, they said there were three things to factor in: the department's needs, the university's needs, and [my] needs. They agreed to make some accommodation for me in compliance with the ADA. However, in my mind, they tried and failed. So eventually, I gave up trying to get accommodations for research and teaching, and I retired from the university. My wife and I asked Dr. Davis, who was very familiar with the details of my recovery, to write a letter about the accommodations I needed so that I could continue to teach.

[The following is a letter sent to the university in support of accommodations to ensure Michael could continue to teach.]

Dear ——,

I have worked with Michael Maher at the University Medical Center for over 2 years. I was chief of the Speech Pathology Department for 27 years and have published scholarly work on the recovery from aphasia, apraxia and alexia. As such, my experience with stroke individuals and directly with Michael gives me confidence that I can provide advice on his case.

Michael has made a dramatic recovery since his stroke 3 years ago. He is by far one of the highest functioning individuals that I have had the pleasure of working with in my 30 years at UCDMC.

Over the past two years, Michael has successfully taught two classes in various locations, in Davis, Sacramento and San Ramon. He found that he needed accommodations and thus asked for the assistance of his wife to ensure that his limitations had not affected his students or performance.

He has asked me to explain his limitations and to recommend accommodations in order for him to continue teaching successfully. His limitations, from my perspective, are the following:

---

16 The ADA is the Americans with Disabilities Act.

Michael has peripheral alexia, which means he has visual deficits that affect his reading. He manages this with intentional eye movements to the right to obviate the visual field cut. He also has a central alexia due to language problems that result in requiring him a slightly longer time to read, process and comprehend written material. He has very mild anomia, which is often indiscernible. Michael requires slightly more time to formulate sentences and prepare arguments so that he uses the words he intends.

Accommodations are as follows: Michael needs support to continue to teach successfully. He needs a dependable individual who is skilled at editing his written work and proofread students' materials returned to him. One suggestion that could be a win-win is to offer a UCD Master level education student, who is interested in alexia/dyslexia, a real-life experience with an individual such as Michael. This student could offer Michael support throughout the quarter in editing and proofreading and in lieu, the student could obtain independent study units or internship credits for working with Michael.

As a professor who has spent her career with individuals with disabilities, I would like to offer why it benefits the university to support Michael. Firstly, it is ethically responsible to make modest accommodations for a tenured professor who has served 28 years at the university as a teacher, scholar and associate dean of faculty. It is a beneficial and unselfish exercise for faculty to make space for their colleague so that he can continue to serve the university and its students to his fullest capacity. There is an intrinsic value to making space for individuals with disabilities in our institutions. Secondly, it serves the students. Michael has already proven to be a successful teacher since his stroke as he has obtained 4.2/5 scores and more "excellent" than "very good" on student evaluations. Lastly, Michael is a true role model to his fellow stroke survivors. They know that he continues to teach, even though it has been challenging, and this has provided them with a successful role model. These modest accommodations are not costly nor do they create an undue burden on the institution and it allows us to keep a valuable resource, Michael.

Respectfully,
Christine Davis PhD
Professor Physical Medicine and Rehabilitation
University of California Davis, Medical Center

What lessons could you pass on to family members or caregivers because of your stroke?
First and foremost, to deal with the medical profession and insurance companies requires an advocate. As a lawyer and CPA, my wife, Kathleen, was a great advocate. My neighbor once said, "Everybody should have a Kathleen!"

Second, be patient with yourself, your family, and your friends, and they must be patient with you. Nobody who hasn't suffered a stroke knows what it is like [to] have a stroke or what it is like for you to encounter the "new you" day in and day out, month after month, and year after year. (I wonder, does it ever get easier?)

Third, don't be too hard on yourself. I'm at about a fifth-grade level in reading, writing, and arithmetic—the three Rs! I encounter the new me every time I do, or try to do, something.

Fourth, find a support group, and/or have your family members also find a support group that meets at least every week. These groups really do help you accomplish reading, writing, and math in a way you cannot do by yourself. In addition, as you support others in your group, they support you.

Fifth, I could not have made so much progress without the help of my dear friends Arnold and Richard. Both visited me often. They were both retired, and it was easy for them to take their time with me. It was a lot of fun. Arnold helped me read and put words into sentences. Richard helped me with word-finding puzzles, proofread my course notes and lecture notes.

What do you think precipitated your stroke?
I think many things, including hereditary factors. My grandfather and father had strokes, but they were much older than me. There were the stresses of

work. In November 2011, the university was targeted by protesters, partially due to tuition hikes. Many departments at the university were shut down, including the business school. I felt like I was at Checkpoint Charlie. I was in charge of the business school while the dean was away taking care of his wife, who had open-heart surgery. I was advised to remove art from the inside of the business school building because the art was loaned from a collection. I guarded the business school from students complaining about tuition increases. It was a stressful time, and I was too busy with the associate dean's job. So I didn't go to see the doctor for my annual physical.

Writing Samples Pre- and Poststroke

This is a note written by Michael the day prior to his stroke.

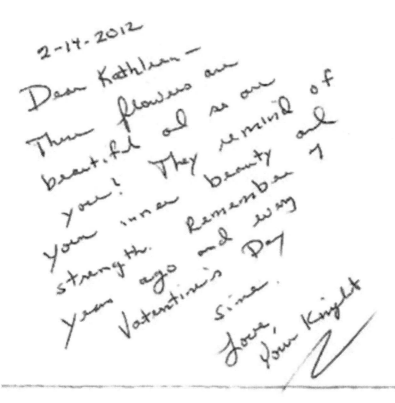

This is Michael's first attempt at writing his name after his stroke.

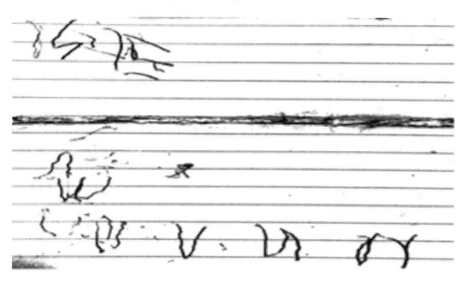

Commentary

Michael's academic success, publications, and textbooks belie a bleak beginning. He was abandoned by his mother and lived with his father and grandparents, who were hardened by ranch life in Idaho. He was raised on a ranch far from town, with few modern conveniences. He has little affection as he looks back on the upbringing he had with his father and grandparents.

He is very close to his two daughters and is proud of his new title of grandfather. He recently said, "I'm glad I had a stroke. I was left with the responsibility of the business department at a difficult time, when there were student demonstrations and an occupation on campus, which was threatening the business school. The school was in the national news for a pepper spray incident of students occupying the campus nonviolently. These events were very stressful and occurred just before my stroke." Michael concludes by saying, "The stroke got me out of the dean's office," and that is not said jokingly.

Michael and his family have found that humor is good medicine. For example, when Michael goes out to dinner with his family and gets tired, he'll announce, "I'm going to take a cab back." His wife remarks, "That's his stroke talking." His stepdaughter adds, "He's a stroke opportunist." And Michael's staff at the university say to him, "You played that stroke card before." Michael recalls these quips fondly.

Final Thoughts

Michael's brain scan is associated with relatively minor language problems. However, in high-achieving individuals like Michael, a little damage to the neural network that supports language can have large and devastating effects. In the fast-paced academic setting, slowed sentence formation and word-finding problems can hinder the progress of one's career.

Today

After retirement Michael continues to write textbooks with his colleagues and with the help of voice-activation software. He used to work with power tools but doesn't trust himself now. Ladders are dicey. He doesn't even use a lawnmower.

Although he claims to be functioning at a fifth- or sixth-grade level, on recent standardized tests, he scored in the college range in vocabulary and reading comprehension. He no longer skis or swims but still dances. He is beginning to pick up the guitar again. He travels with his wife and solo to see his children and grandchildren in Colorado and New Zealand. He drives independently and has balance issues but otherwise no physical disabilities. He is engaged socially and enjoys going to lunch with his friends, singly rather than in groups. He says, "It's easier to follow the conversation."

Michael's Brain Scan[17]

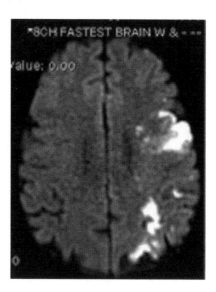

---

17 White areas on the image indicate damage on the left side of brain. Michael's brain scan is consistent with relatively minor language problems.

Michael's Wife, Kathleen: Thoughts on the Stroke

Tell us what happened at the time of your husband's stroke.

It was Wednesday, February 15, 2012. As I look back on the early morning that Michael experienced his stroke, I try not to dwell on the ways I feel I failed him. I feel my first mistake was not recognizing the signs of a stroke. Michael woke me by standing over me, gently shaking me, and forming the only sound available to him: a guttural grunt. Michael's only symptom was that he could not form words. In every other respect, he seemed completely himself. He was physically OK. He was communicating with me through body language. He seemed cognitively OK. But he was not; he was experiencing a major stroke event.

If you are reading this, it may be because someone you know has had a stroke or you have had a stroke yourself. If you didn't know the signs of a stroke, as I did not, it's not too late to help teach others the signs to be aware of: inability to speak or slurred speech, droopy face or inability to smile, and paralysis or inability to lift either arm for more than a second or two. (The mnemonic is FAST, as in "act fast": face droop, arm weakness, speech slurred or strange, time to call 911.)

What did you do at the time?

I didn't know what exactly was wrong with my husband, but I knew we needed help. Although he was mobile, walking, and even dressing himself to go to the hospital, I knew in my heart something really serious was happening. We got to the hospital, and we received the news fairly quickly. The doctor said, "You have had a stroke. The only thing left to do is recover."

The question of tPA came up.[18] While we were trying to communicate with Michael and find out when the stroke began, I made my first mistake as an advocate for him: I let an emergency-room volunteer silence me while I was trying to probe Michael and perhaps get some clue as to when the stroke began. I had some hints, but I was not going to take a chance, as the doctor told us tPA can be fatal if administered outside the three-hour window of the onset of the stroke.

---

18 tPA is tissue plasminogen activator, a protein that helps break down blood clots.

What did you learn at this stage that may be useful to others in your situation?
Please take this advice to heart: every stroke survivor needs an advocate in the hospital and at all times, if possible! Michael and I both witnessed the level of care administered to patients who were alone and had nobody to speak up for them. I rarely left my husband's side after his stroke. He got the best possible care from his medical team because I demanded it—and almost always in a kind and professional way. When that way didn't work, I had to become more convincing and demanding. The need for advocacy did not end when we left the hospital; it did not end after we left the rehabilitation center; it has not ended yet.

Did he have therapies?
My husband was fortunate to have the speech, physical, and occupational therapy he needed after he returned home. I attended every single therapy session so I could replicate at home what the therapists were doing with Michael during their time with him.

I didn't know stroke recovery was difficult and didn't always work to the patient's expectation. I had no experience in this area. So, when we set a goal that Michael would return to work after a year of therapy and recovery, there was nothing left to do but help him meet that goal. We worked very hard together, but Michael's success is a result of the fact that he never gave up trying. He began working on recovery his first night in the hospital, Wednesday. I was lying on a hospital chair that turned into a bed and looking at him between hospital-bed rails. With his left hand, he was prying open each finger of his now-crippled right hand. By the time he got through his entire hand, the fingers were curled up again, but that didn't stop him from trying again and again.

How were you feeling during this time?
Our positive mind-sets and hopeful expectations carried us through most of the first year of recovery. I never doubted that my husband would return to work. He had doubts, I know now, but he never shared them with me. Next

piece of advice: make sure your loved one has an outlet where he can express his darkest fears or where she can complain about how difficult recovery is.

During Michael's rehabilitation, speech, occupational, and physical therapists, counselors, doctors, and friends all asked about how I was doing. "Are you taking time for yourself? Are you practicing self-care?" Every time I was asked, I got defensive and angry. This was not about me; it was about my husband. I didn't want to practice self-care. I wanted to help my husband heal. I now know I was wrong to think that. I paid a big price later.

What advice would you give to those who, like you, are the spouse of a stroke survivor?
My next piece of advice is to take some time—all the time you need—to keep yourself healthy and happy and not feel guilty about it. If you don't, it may come back to haunt you, as it did me. That old cliché is true: you can't take care of anyone else if you don't care for yourself first.

I isolated myself from my friends and family because caring for my husband was a full-time job (or so I told myself). I didn't spend any time enjoying myself, because Michael was working so hard at recovery. Who was I to simply be carrying on with my life as it was before? It felt disloyal to have fun, be with friends, and live my life.

How did you get through this?
About three and a half years after Michael's stroke, I started really coming apart at the seams. I had yet to deal with the loss I experienced and the ways my life changed after his stroke. I went through most of the stages of grief at that point: denial/isolation, anger, bargaining with my higher power, depression, and acceptance (which I'm still working on). I learned it is OK to grieve. We who are affected by a loved one's stroke must grieve and not feel guilty about it.

Initially, whenever I started to grieve, I would berate myself: "How dare you feel sorry for yourself? Michael had the stroke, not you! You can still speak and read and write and type and do everything you could do before." Then I would stuff down those feelings or feel guilty for even considering my loss.

But I learned to acknowledge I have experienced loss too. The Michael I fell in love with and married and spent eight wonderful years with was very different from the Michael I now lived with. We no longer communicated as before. Many conversations ended in misunderstanding or frustration. I sought help from a counselor. Her advice ultimately was this: "Your entire life before was intertwined with Michael's life. You must learn to have some of your life apart from his now." I didn't want to accept that, but I knew she was right.

Did your life change after his stroke?
We didn't do many of the same activities together anymore. Physical changes in Michael made it difficult. Our counselor told me, "You must develop your own interests and seek support in your friends and family to enjoy those activities again." Again, she was right. Before my husband's stroke, I know, I was very lucky to have an extremely loving, caring, unselfish, and successful man who made all my dreams come true. Most of us never get that, even for one day. I honestly felt like a little girl who woke up one day and had become a princess.

This brings me to another topic: attitude. After Michael's stroke, my attitude was optimistic. I'm an optimist by nature. I was optimistic he would recover, we would get adequate medical care, our friends and family would adjust, and life would return to nearly normal if we worked hard enough at it. Michael made such tremendous gains in the first year. He made additional gains the next year. But I didn't know how to temper my expectations for recovery. Every stroke survivor is different. Every recovery is different. My attitude now is "This is where we are now. Now is all there really is, so let's live here." When we aren't mourning the past or fearing the future, life is pretty darn good.

I also didn't know how Michael was dealing with the stroke. He was the strong, silent type. He just kept working at it. He still works at it. I advise you as the support person to let your stroke survivor know it is OK to let his or her body heal in its own time, not on anyone else's schedule.

What is your final bit of advice?

Finally, if you, your family, and your stroke survivor didn't have a healthy sense of humor before the stroke, now might be a good time to try to develop one. After Michael's stroke, people used the term *stroke victim* to characterize him. I refused to allow that. So, we mostly used the term *stroke survivor*. But my daughter Emily found a humorous term for whenever Michael's stroke gave him an advantage in how he was treated or in getting his way in a family decision: *stroke opportunist!* We still joke about that to this day whenever Michael, although outnumbered in the family vote, gets his way.

Today

Kathleen is a former decorated athlete and marathon runner. She is in private practice as a tax attorney and loves her work. She is actively involved in her alumni association, has numerous friends, travels, and is a loving mother to her children.

Michael's Daughter Kai

How were you first notified about your father's stroke?
I was a lawyer and taking a deposition at the time. I got a call from my stepmom, Kathleen. I picked up the phone, and I can't remember exactly what she said, but I told her I would call her back. She sounded a little anxious. I thought maybe something had happened to my mom. My mom lived in Davis, and my dad and Kathleen helped me keep an eye on her because she was having health issues.

I called Kathleen back, and she told me my dad had a stroke. It was the last thing I expected to hear. I was in California the weekend before his stroke, and I had the chance to spend time with him while he drove me from Napa to Sacramento. I had never seen him so stressed out and feeling negative about work. He has always been positive.

My dad's family tends to live for a long time. His dad had a stroke in his seventies. I just assumed my dad was healthy. I did not expect that something like this was going to happen. At the time, I was living in Denver, and I left everything and took a plane to California.

Can you remember any of the feelings you had?
I was in the moment, so I had to go through the motions. I knew I had to get my plane ticket and assess what I needed to do at work before I left.

I don't remember the details Kathleen told me, but I knew he was alive and his brain was affected. Kathleen said my dad walked down the stairs at home. By the time they got to the hospital, his right side started to get worse.

When I got there, my dad had already had a bad experience when he panicked in the MRI. Kathleen was very protective, so she was horrified about the whole thing. It was clear he was pretty traumatized.

What did he tell you was stressful for him about his work?
The students were protesting tuition hikes, and the campus police peppersprayed the students—it was in the national news—and that was stressful. He taught in the business school at UC Davis. I knew some of his students because

I went to law school at UC Davis. I heard from peers that they loved my father as a professor. I knew he took it very seriously and took it to heart when people had massive complaints they took to him as he was in a leadership position. That was really hard on him even though he couldn't do much about it.

He was also having problems with his publisher. I don't know what the exact situation was, but since the stroke I have had a different perspective on publishing. I get that they are in the business of making money, but he had a stroke, and they were still interested only in the bottom line. Before that weekend, I had never really heard my dad talk about being stressed at work, but this was different. I could tell he was really stressed, because he was talking about it so much. He was also teaching an extra class, which could have been stressful too.

Kathleen was studying for the bar exam. My stepsister, Kathleen's daughter, was graduating from high school, and Kathleen was very concerned about her as well.

What happened when you got to Sacramento?
My stepsister picked me up from the airport, and we went to the hospital. I remember seeing Kathleen and bursting into tears, and we hugged each other. Dad still looked like himself. He did not have any facial drooping, but the look in his eyes was different. He just looked so far away. He was clearly not feeling like himself. He is usually hardworking and manages his stuff pretty easily; he's smart and very positive and a very verbal person. We used to laugh at how long his voice messages were. I hadn't seen him with any health conditions before. It was hard to see him in a hospital bed and in a gown. I think he knew I was there. I felt he was glad I was there. But everything was shocking. I kept thinking how it must have been for Kathleen taking Dad to the hospital.

How did he communicate with you?
I know that at some point he was mumbling something. No actual words were coming out of his mouth. He would squeeze my hand. One day he took my hand and patted me. I think he felt bad about how stressful it was for me. Who knows whether it was just all in my head? I felt he was telling me he was sorry. He patted my hand and gave me this look. He was so used to being the rock.

The therapist talked to us about his eating. She said to turn his head to one side to help him swallow. It was hard to know what he wanted to eat, because he was not able to talk. Some folks visited, and he would laugh at the things they were saying, but his words were unintelligible. At one point on Thursday, he wanted to say something. I said, "Do you want something to drink?" and he shook his head and mumbled, but he was making a sequence of sounds. So I asked him, "Do you want to go to the bathroom?" and he got more and more frustrated. He kept saying the same jumbled sounds. He got so frustrated that at one point he yelled at me, "No!" He was clearly frustrated and upset, but I was happy he had finally said something. Kathleen and I said, "Oh my God, you said something!"

That Friday Kathleen told me he had said "table" and "love you." They got him to sing some songs, and that was very exciting. It was weird because of what was going on in his brain; it was fascinating. I felt something like adrenaline; I felt very positive as I left the hospital. His recovery was amazing. It's still very impressive.

I sat with him when he had an ultrasound on his neck to locate the clot. It showed a clot in his carotid artery. The doctor told us which part of his brain was affected. She told us it was a massive stroke. As she spoke with us, I was trying to process it, and I asked questions. I let things sink in. It had affected a lot of his brain. I was processing that, but I was also amazed. I was affected by his recovery and the fact that Kathleen had saved my dad's life. She had her act together and did what was right for my dad. That has affected how I see relationships.

Kathleen thought about postponing taking the bar exam. I told her she needed to take it. She had studied for it, and it was such a stressor for the family. I told her she had to just take it. I knew she was very well prepared. Turns out that was the right decision.

Dad was very supportive and helped her through law school. I remember Kathleen saying he had been carrying all the weight for them and now she would carry all the weight for the family. I think this was huge, and the dynamic of the relationship changed. She didn't realize she was going through something traumatic. She took on a mothering role, trying to protect him even with visitors.

I kept feeling an adrenaline rush. I have talked with friends that have had similar experiences. I don't know whether it has to do with being close to a life-threatening situation or the hope for recovery. I experienced positivity and a sort of high for a couple of days.

You are having all these insights about Kathleen. Did you ever tell her about them?
I remember telling her she was going through something traumatic and she needed to acknowledge and accept that [the stroke] had changed her as well. Dad had always paid a lot of attention to her before his stroke. But now she felt that whenever she walked into a room where he was, he would not even notice she was there. I thought it was his brain and he couldn't help it. It was a change from how it was before to suddenly feeling as if he was not noticing her.

Are you worried about them?
I noticed those things at the beginning, and over the years since it happened, I have worried a lot. It's probably not fair to them, because they had a very awesome relationship. I thought that was what a marriage should be like. It has been very scary at times, how things have changed and how their dynamic has changed. They are still really sweet to each other, but they have been through some rough patches.

How has your relationship with your dad changed?
I feel that in a lot of ways, he mellowed. There was some tension in our relationship, but that has gone away since his stroke. I feel we are in a good place. Since his stroke, Dad jokes around. For instance, [to get his way], he'll say, "I'm playing the stroke card." It seems he has a really good attitude. He takes a Zen approach to everything.

Was he that way before?
He had a piece of it in some ways; he was always pretty mellow. He was the type of person who would not bother about the little things. But as I said, he was very stressed before his stroke. Dad is now a Zen master. He just seems very mellow and has a great attitude about everything. We think it is very cool.

My sister and I talk about it. Definitely his personality had an element of that before, but not to this extent.

He was a very high-functioning person; he was a professor, and there is a type of stress that goes with that. He had an element of "yeah, whatever." I think it kicked up after his stroke. I believe it helps him cope with the stroke. I think he is a very positive person and he never wants conflicts. He likes to keep things light and positive and likes to joke. I have heard him say he is a stroke opportunist. Maybe that originated with him. I think it's clever.

How are you processing the relationship with your dad?
I think for a while I had this weird feeling because I missed my old dad, but then I was so happy about how positive my dad seemed after the stroke. It is sort of confusing because I feel as if Dad is gone in some ways but not really gone. His personality fundamentally did not change. I know that some people can be affected that way by strokes. He communicates more, and we have this great relationship. For example, my husband and my sister's partner met Dad after his stroke. They know him just as he is now. They both say they don't notice when he is struggling with words or language, as my sister and I do.

I worry about whether people are treating him right. I know Kathleen is protective of him, maybe too much so, but at the same time, I completely understand why. For example, two weeks after he got out of the hospital, we went to the movies, and he ordered popcorn. He didn't use a lot of words to order the popcorn, so the clerk took the lead. I was watching him as he ordered, and I felt very protective of him. I saw how the clerk reacted to my dad and was wondering whether he would be nice. I don't think the clerk even noticed anything. I was just very protective, and I didn't want anyone to make my dad feel bad. Dad was cool with it all.

So I still feel kind of worried about how vulnerable he is. I know that at school, he had some tense conversations with his colleagues. I felt very worried about whether he was articulating what he wanted and whether he was able to represent himself and his interests. Is he able to advocate for himself without being easily influenced by what other people want? That is what I worry about.

What advice would you give to daughters and sons of stroke survivors?
I was very glad I was there with him. My words of wisdom would be to be there. It sounds simple, but just do that. It can be scary, but it does feel amazing. There are many amazing things. You just realize that many things can change literally overnight. That is pretty upsetting sometimes, but you try to be there. You adjust.

Be there for your parent who had a stroke. For example, Dad has thanked me for letting him say what he wanted to say. He told me others would try to jump in and try to say what he wanted to say for him.

I would ask his therapists what I could do to help so I could help him with his homework. I tried to contribute to his recovery. I had experience tutoring kids, so I coped by trying to help. Talking to people about strokes and learning about it was pretty comforting. Dad is a very hardworking person, and he worked very hard at his recovery.

Today

Kai works as an attorney and loves her work. She is a new mother and devoted daughter to her father. Michael often drives or flies to Denver to visit his daughter and new grandson.

Emily, Michael's Stepdaughter

Tell us about the event of Michael's stroke.
The night before was Valentine's Day, and all three of us—Michael, my mom, and I—had dinner together. The next morning, I woke up very late for high school. I was a senior, graduating in just a few months. Admittedly, I was annoyed that no one had made sure I was awake. I was even more annoyed when I discovered that not only was everyone gone but the car I was planning on driving that day was gone too. I didn't think anything could possibly be wrong. My mom called me right as my last class of the day was about to begin, asking me to come outside to talk. My initial thought was that I was in trouble, and as I walked down the stairs to the front of the school, I tried to think of what I could possibly have done. When I got to the car, I noticed that my mom seemed very detached, which is very atypical of her. "Emily, Michael had a stroke. He's going to be OK, though. And he's going to recover." I think she was trying to convince herself more than she was trying to reassure me. I wasn't really sure how to respond. I knew it was bad; I knew what a stroke was. But I couldn't possibly have imagined how it would affect our lives. My mom asked me to come to the hospital after class. I didn't immediately react. I responded with an OK, a hug, and a promise to see her soon.

How were you feeling at that time?
I walked back to my class but sat outside the door first. That was when the severity of the situation hit me, and I immediately felt guilty. As a teenager, I wasn't the easiest to tolerate. I took a lot of personal issues out on Michael, and I thought I was entirely to blame for his stroke, that I was the sole stressor in his life. I even felt guilty for being so frustrated that morning about the car, when the reason it was gone was that my mom was driving Michael to the hospital. I felt selfish and angry. It took me some time to compose myself, but eventually I was able to calm down enough to return to class.

What was it like when you first saw Michael in the hospital?
When I arrived at the hospital after school, I didn't know what to expect. I followed my mom to Michael's room and prepared myself. But I could not have

prepared myself for what I saw. There lay one of the smartest men I knew, unable to even say the word "me." The most composed, gentle man I knew was kicking and crying in a hospital bed. That was the first time I ever saw Michael upset, and whenever I try to understand what he must have been feeling—the fear, the anger, the frustration—my heart breaks all over again.

How did this affect your life?
In a sense, I was presented with two choices when Michael had his stroke: consider myself helpless and do nothing, or step up and do what I could to help. However, it was never a choice for me. There was no question that I'd choose the second option. The next few weeks, I did whatever I needed to do to keep the household in order. Throughout the weeks following Michael's stroke, I tried to make life easier for my mom. I took care of our two dogs. While my friends were out having fun, celebrating, and preparing for graduation, I was at the rehabilitation center where my stepdad was a patient. If I wasn't there, delivering clean clothes to my mom or making sure she was eating, I was at home studying or doing homework.

Family friends flooded us with an abundance of food. It was incredible and generous and relieved one more responsibility in our lives. But slowly, we started getting only a few meals a week, and eventually they stopped altogether. People had to continue with their lives, including our family. I had prom and graduation ahead. There were bills to pay, dogs to feed, and meals to cook.

How did this affect your relationship?
I assumed everything would be the same as before. I think it's typical to expect things to return to how they were before a stroke in the family, to expect that everyone and everything will go back to normal. But I think it's these expectations that hurt everyone more than they helped. People in all aspects of Michael's life placed enormous expectations on him, especially him. And I'll be the first to admit that my expectations weren't entirely realistic. I saw him progress rapidly, and I kept pushing him forward—actually, I would say I pushed him backward, toward our previous lifestyle. I did this out of love, because I truly thought he was going to make a full recovery. But instead, I feel

I pushed him away. I think the most important thing to accept is that the old normal isn't going to be the norm anymore. But instead of fighting against the current situation, you have to normalize it, make it the new normal. This is a notion I'm still trying to accept, all these years later. I find myself expecting behaviors from Michael that just aren't feasible for him anymore. If I could go back and give myself advice from the beginning, it would be not to take anything he does or says personally. Finding offense in things that are sometimes out of his control after the stroke, I've only set our relationship up to deteriorate. Sometimes I confront him about these behaviors. Seeing the pain, he feels for hurting me or others close to him, I realize they aren't intentional. I know Michael experiences frustration, depression, and anxiety still, and I've noticed his pride continues to be important to him. As someone who loves and cares about Michael, I want to help ameliorate these feelings, not aggravate them. I don't let his stroke be an excuse for some of the hurt he causes me, but I have learned I don't have to hold him accountable for *everything*.

Do you have advice for others in your situation?
Looking back on the past years, I see there were plenty of opportunities for me to do something different, something better. But after you experience a stroke in the family, all you can do is the best you can. Open, honest communication is so important. So is acceptance. I'm continually reminding myself there are no "should haves" after this experience, because that only leads to guilt. For me, there are no "could laters," because that only leads to anxiety. Instead, I have found it's possible only to support one another in the present, as best as we can.

Five

THE QUARTERBACK: I'M TOO YOUNG TO HAVE A STROKE!

Jason was a college quarterback and is still built like one. He humbly states he wasn't the starting quarterback. By his own admission, he is shy. Before his stroke, he was a coach for middle school basketball and high school football. He loved the kids. It was there at school he had his stroke at age forty-three.

Jason is dedicated to his family. When asked, he brags about his nine-year-old daughter, Abby, who is a talented singer. He is amazed by the fact that months after his stroke, he and his wife became pregnant with Cass. This was after trying for years to have a second child.

Jason is one of the youngest in our group. He has had emotional lability and easily cries, especially when speaking about his family. He expresses himself in fits and starts. In language activities in the group, he is stellar at unscrambling letters to form words, spelling, word-finding puzzles, and virtually any task that requires reading. His only trouble is with fluency, such as talking spontaneously. He also has right hemiparesis of both his arm and leg, but he can walk independently with a limp. A year after his stroke, he walked three miles with his friend in a fundraiser to raise awareness for stroke. He regained his license and retrofitted his truck so the brake and accelerator could be operated by the left foot. This increased not only his independence but also his self-esteem.

Here is his story.

What do you remember about the stroke?
I was playing basketball. In second period, I took a shot, but it was short. That was pretty unusual for me. So I walked back to the office. I couldn't talk. I really didn't know what to do. I went back into the gym, and I couldn't talk at all.

Did you limp?
No, I just couldn't talk, and I went all day, and nobody noticed. I couldn't talk to take roll. So I went out to practice. I was coaching a bunch of boys; I couldn't tell them to go run or anything.

Were the kids looking at you kind of funny?
Yes. The other coach said to go to the hospital. My friend drove me to the emergency room. He couldn't understand what was going on. He couldn't understand me. In the emergency room, they left me on the table. I thought, "I am not going to stand for this kind of treatment." The doctors were there, but for another six hours, they didn't do anything.

I stayed at Kaiser Hospital another night. They were going to discharge me. I went to the bathroom, and it was there that I fell and had another stroke. This more severely injured my body, my right side. Then they wanted me to go home, and my wife said, "Wait, you need to give him another day." She found me a place in San Francisco, and I was there for four weeks. It was a rehab place in San Francisco, not part of Kaiser. They fitted me with a brace, but they did not really help with arm exercises.

What about the speech therapist?
It was good, but the amount of work she made me do was too much, you know. She was asking me to do way more than what I was able to do. Four weeks in San Francisco, and then they said I can go home.

What were you thinking while you were in rehab?

I was scared. I was not familiar with aphasia, and my mind was going at a hundred miles per hour. They got me a wheelchair. I did not like that very much. My mom and dad were there.

Did your parents help?

I don't think so. I don't think my parents understood. I don't think that it would have helped if they understood. We went home, and my wife was really trying to push for me. Then she found a rehab center in Dallas. I was there for two weeks. They put me in this machine; it was going opposite and sideways. It was going around and around, and I did that for two weeks. We went for one more time two weeks after that for a refresher.

How did you hear about the university program?

My wife got me into UC Davis. I was here in the outpatient clinic for four months. I saw Ryan for physical therapy. I saw speech therapy, and I have done Sentence Structure Group.

What are your biggest challenges now?

I don't know. I kind of have my marriage and my kids. We were trying to conceive a child. My wife could not adjust to the fact that we couldn't have a second child. Then I had the stroke, and we had a baby. I think my wife is happy.

What are you hoping for yourself?

I hope my marriage works out. We have had countless hours of therapy. I am not a big fan of therapy, but our therapist is good. The therapist gets my wife to talk about our needs and wants. My wife is at a different level than I am. I am right down here, and she is way up there. She has more ability to explain herself. I can't bring my thoughts on paper or in a session. I can't come close to explaining myself.

What is your role at home?

I got my car back. I am driving, and I am independent at home. I set the table, wash dishes, and cook. I landscape sometimes. Sylvia, our housekeeper, comes every two weeks. Kathy, the babysitter, works with our daughter Cass. Cass is not really talking, so Kathy works with her.

Have you found a support group?
I like it, not that much. I found a group at Rancho Cordova. I had lunch with a woman who was also affected by the same kind of stroke. I met with her in Rancho Cordova with other people who have had strokes. I met Michael, and I talked to him for about an hour. Michael talks good, but he is way younger. At twenty-five years old, he had a stroke eight years ago. Dorsi, who is forty-three, had a full stroke, and she reads braille. She had a stroke like mine, but she has her language all together.

What are your thoughts about where you are now?
It has been two and a half years. I see the world different now. I've got my friend John, and the rest are not around me and haven't explained themselves to me. I see John once a month. I go to his house. I can talk to him about everything. We have a lot to share.

Do you have siblings?
I just went to Colorado to see my brother, Rob. It was perfect. I went to see Ragen [Rob's daughter]. She is at the University of Wyoming. I would hang out with her and watch her do her running events. I would also go watch her younger brother, Hyden; he is fifteen.

It seems you have a good relationship with your brother. Tell me about your parents.
My dad is still going strong, and my mom is slowly winding down.

Do you keep working on your speech?
I am reading with Cass, and I am reading pretty fluently. Cass is a year and seven months. She has some words. Kathy is there to help her with her development.

How is your relationship with your oldest daughter?
She is singing. I admire her. She is doing great at school.

Is there anything you have learned from your stroke?
I think it is too early to talk about what I've learned.

Commentary

Jason is the only member of our group who now works. He is pretty pleased he got a job with the local baseball team pitching whiffle balls and working the two-man slides and the trampoline for the kids. Jason has anomic aphasia, primarily word-finding problems, and he has great potential. It is very likely he will have better facility of spontaneous speech in the future.

Fortunately for Jason, his wife has been a tireless advocate for him. She saw that Stanford had published about their success injecting stem cells into the brains of stroke survivors to treat deficits. She contacted Stanford and now has Jason enlisted for prescreening in this research trial.

Today

Jason is working for the local baseball team. He drives independently even as far as Wyoming and Colorado to see his brothers and his niece and nephew. He is a devoted father. But by his own admission, he is still not where he wants to be.

Carla, Jason's Mother

Tell me a little bit about how you heard your son had a stroke.
We were at home and got a phone call. The coaches from the high school took Jason to the hospital. Someone suggested it would be helpful if we took care of Abby, Jason's daughter, so his wife could go to the hospital. We drove up and understood the doctors were running tests. We thought he got hurt at work.

So we got Abby. When we heard it could have been a stroke, we thought, "No way. He is too young. Must be another issue." I didn't realize it until the next morning. His wife was with her brother at the hospital. We heard Jason had a slight stroke and stroked again in the morning when he fell in the bathroom. That is the one that hit him hard. He was released and went to San Francisco for rehabilitation.

How was Jason doing?
He was frustrated. He couldn't get a thought out of his mouth. At four weeks, he was released and walked with a cane. His speech was not good.

He came home, and a gentleman came three times a week. His wife did a lot of exercises with his arm and leg, about an hour a day. I worked with him on his speech. I chatted with him and did worksheets, like opposites, first- to second-grade materials. He was shut down with the whole process.

But he surprised me. He did word scrambles, Sudoku. His brain worked better than he could say. I'm a great puzzle person, but he would finish them for me. I encouraged him by saying, "You're better than me." After one month, his wife took him to Texas, and we stayed with Abby. Once he found out his arm wasn't coming back, he was bummed and lost all hope.

What was Jason like growing up?
He's been a quiet young man all his life, well liked and smart. He was not outgoing. He was so well liked he had friends constantly. His friends all came to him. He was reserved. He did not initiate. He was happy to be by himself.

How were his spirits?

Once Jason started driving again, it was a saving grace. It boosted his self-esteem. He went to Colorado to be with his brother. There he couldn't think of a word he wanted to say. He remembered it at two in the morning: "*Elk*, it's *elk!*" His brother and his kids are great with him. He has a special relationship with Hyden, who is athletic.

How did Jason's children adjust?

Abby is fine with her dad. At first she was standoffish, but now she is good and loving. She'll say, "Come on, Dad. Play dominos." She is very talented.

How do you feel about his recovery?

We are pretty happy. We understood that you could recover up to seven years. He feels he is getting better too.

Bob, Jason's Father

What were your first thoughts when Jason had his stroke?
First thing I thought was that he was so young. It can happen to anyone. My dad was in his sixties when he had a stroke. My advice is to have medical checkups.

How did you help your son?
I tried to work with him, keep his morale up. He is a "my way or no way" kind of guy. I tried to give him something to do; for example, we would hang a bulletin board or put a bed together. I tried to keep him going so he wouldn't get bummed out. I was born and raised on a dairy farm. We worked hard. So that is how I helped him. I encouraged him to help out. I would say, "Come on, Jason. We're going to plant a tree." I encouraged him to help. It would make him feel good about himself.

Did he improve?
He has improved a lot. [But] he is 50 percent of where he should be.

He perked up when he drove. He is more independent. The gas pedal was moved to the left side, by the brake. He uses his left leg for the gas and brake. We went to baseball games, and he would say, "I'm driving, Dad." He has slowed down a lot and is a more cautious driver. He even tells me, "Dad, slow down!"

What advice would you give others?
It is a matter of being patient and kind. Let them take care of things. Give them an open door to vent feelings. Love them and expect more and more.

Six

A Husband's Perspective

*J*eff gives us his point of view as the spouse of Jana, a successful ombudsman for the state of California. She had warning signs of an impending stroke, but they were misdiagnosed as medication side effects.

Did your wife have any signs before her stroke?
Jana had a time, about six weeks, when she had really low energy, and that was very unusual for her since she was a high-energy person. We went to the doctor a couple of times and thought she had a vitamin deficiency or something like that, but they couldn't find anything. That was the only indication that something was going on. She was fifty-three at the time.

What happened when she had the stroke? Were you there?
I was not. I was at work, and she had taken time off from work because she didn't feel well enough to go. She called me and said, "I got an e-mail from my friend Gail, and I can't understand the e-mail." I told her to read me the e-mail, and although she could speak well, she was reading gibberish. So I told her to spell it for me and things like that. I told her I was going to go home and we were going to go to the ER.

I think she'd been having the stroke. I think the blood vessel broke a day or two before she called me at work and things had gotten progressively worse after we went to the doctor. There was no event that indicated all of a sudden that she had had a stroke. She just had the cognitive issues and the speech issues.[19]

Do you remember when it occurred?
It was around the first week of August on a Friday. We went to the doctor's office because the doctor had given her a new prescription for her exhaustion. But on Monday he said not to take the medicine anymore, because of her confusion. The next day, she called me about the e-mail. That was the day we went to the ER and they did a bunch of tests. They suspected it was a thrombosis in her left jugular vein.

What were you feeling when this was happening?
Well, there was a lot of fear. There was a lot of wonder and confusion in terms of wondering what was going to happen to my wife and whether they were going to figure out what it was. Then they were talking about a stroke and possible brain surgery. It was a time of great emotional turmoil. I don't know whether that adequately captures my feelings at the time.

Did she go into surgery?
No, the neurosurgeon came in and said she was not a neurosurgery candidate but they could use drugs that would coagulate the blood rather than surgery.

How long was she in the hospital?
For two weeks.

Did you think she was at risk for severe disability or death?
The doctors did prepare us for that possibility. There was definite concern early on. There was a lot of anxiety and emotion because we didn't know what her recovery would be like.

---

19 These are in fact signs of a stroke.

She could talk, just not very well. She couldn't name things or carry on much of a conversation. They gave her that test where they show you a picture and you tell them what's going on. She could name some things, but she couldn't say a continuous sentence. They came and did that every couple of hours.

Did she have any physical signs?
No, just cognitive.

When she was in the hospital, did she have speech therapy?
She did, some. I remember Dr. Christine Davis came in, and that was the first time I met her. We were in the ICU. They assigned a therapist to her when she was in the hospital. When we left, we had to go get speech therapy. We didn't have physical therapy.

Do you think the doctors should have done more when she first came in with symptoms instead of turning her away?
That's a question I've thought about a lot over the years. The practice of medicine is eliminating things to come to a solution. At that time she wasn't presenting as if she had a stroke, so I think it would have taken a very astute doctor to figure out what was going on. Since they had given her a new medication and she was having symptoms that were consistent with the side effects of that medication, they just said to lay off the medication and see how she felt Monday. I don't blame the doctors. I don't think that's productive or even fair. Once they figured out what it was, they gave her great treatment at UC Davis. Do I wish they had figured it out sooner? Sure. I think that could have eliminated some of the damage.

How much time did you take off work?
I took off work the first week she was in the hospital. Then I came and saw her every day before work, during lunchtime, and after work for the rest of her hospital stay. Then when she went home, her parents, who lived close, came and stayed with her. Her mom was a teacher, and she started to help my wife with speech therapy right away.

What did her mother work on with her?

She started back in early grade school lessons, and our friend Cheryl put Post-it notes around the house, like "This is a chair" and "This is a table." Cheryl got some sheets that had pictures of things, and she worked with her on simple spelling and reading. Jana's dad helped her with flash cards. Jay's parents also took her to speech therapy four days a week. One interesting aspect is my wife couldn't read words but she could spell them. I could say, "Spell 'Atlantic Ocean,'" and she would spell it; then I would write it on the lap board, and she couldn't read it. That was an indication for me that the information was still there, just not accessible, which was a glimmer of hope.

How was your wife after her stroke?

She was depressed; she was fearful. She had a lot of anxiety about performing. She would go to a group but not be able to participate, so that created more anxiety.

I've been to group only a couple of times, and there's a wide spectrum of people in the group. I think a group is a way for people to see they're not alone.

Commentary

How did Jana get out of her depression? Her husband simply needed her. Jana's husband was diagnosed with cancer. Jana had been taking antidepressants, but it was a matter of purpose and necessity that motivated her up and out of her depression. His diagnosis forced her to take care of him and thereby leave her depression behind.

Today

Jana had her stroke at fifty-three. She is fully independent. She has no mobility deficits but exhibits infrequent word-finding problems and processing difficulties. She drives and travels with her husband. Her brain scan shows extensive damage from a hemorrhagic stroke. Hemorrhage is less common and accounts for about 15 percent of strokes. Here is another example of how a brain scan does not predict outcome. When interacting with Jana, it is hard to detect that she ever had a stroke!

Jana's Brain Scan on the Right and Normal Brain on the Left[20]

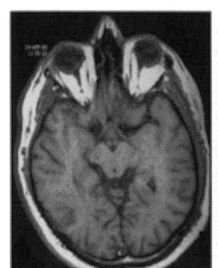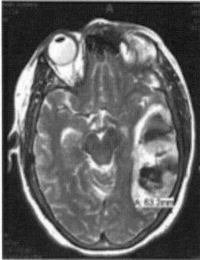

---

20 The scan of Jana's brain, on the right, shows damage from a large intraparenchymal hemorrhage within the left temporal lobe. Intraparenchymal hemorrhage is bleeding within the cerebral hemispheres.

Part II

Broca's Aphasia

Disability is a term that simply means that we need accommodations to participate fully in our society.

—US Board of Equal Opportunity

B roca's aphasia is an expressive aphasia. It is characterized by difficulty finding words and putting words into sentences. Although it is considered an expressive aphasia, that description is not entirely accurate. Individuals with Broca's aphasia also have problems understanding lengthy and complex speech. They have problems with reading and writing as well. The following stories are told by individuals with Broca's aphasia and their families. Becky, Barb, Don, and Mike have Broca's aphasia. Here are their stories.

Seven

BARB: FROM FAST TRACK TO "SLOW DOWN AND SMELL THE ROSES"

Barb is bespectacled and delightful. She had her stroke when she was forty-three years old and has been in the group for seven years. She is petite with an obvious paralysis of her right side, her hand contracted, and a brace on her right leg. She has a cane but rarely needs or uses it. Prior to her stroke, she traveled numerous times to Ubud, Bali, a Hindu spiritual center. She stayed in an ashram long before *Eat, Pray, Love* promoted travel to Bali. Even now she has the aura of someone who has been close to spiritualism. Barb worked for a stockbroker firm in San Francisco and loved the "fast life" but now says she has more time to "smell the roses." Although she is classified as having Broca's aphasia, characterized by telegraphic speech, her vocabulary is abundant. She reads and articulates multisyllabic words well but stumbles on pronouns and prepositions. She can't differentiate those pesky small words, such as *of* from *if* and *they* from *he*, especially while reading. Her greatest difficulty is with numbers. When she was a stock executive, numbers came easy, but now even simple calculations are difficult for Barb.

Here is her story.

Tell us what happened before your stroke.

I was living the good life in San Francisco before my stroke. I had a high-powered job in marketing at Bloomberg with accounts all over the West Coast. At age forty-three, I loved the fast pace of Bloomberg and life in San Francisco. Five days before New Year's 2002, I went to the doctor because I was not feeling well. The interior light in my office was bothering me, and I was having headaches. The doctor sent me home, saying it was a cold or the flu. So I went back to work despite the fact that I was feeling under the weather and my head was throbbing.

When did you have the stroke?

It was on New Year's Eve 2002. I was at home on the computer. Suddenly, I got dizzy and collapsed. I was in and out of consciousness for a whole day with only Smoky, my cat, to comfort me. I learned later that I received calls from my friend Cindy; my brother, Mike; and my sister, Pam. But I wasn't able to answer the phone. I spent the next twenty-four hours lying on the floor of my apartment. I hoped that someone would find me before I died.

After you woke up, what happened?

I thought about my sister and brother and hoped they would come help me. One day later, Pam from Santa Rosa and Mike came in, because they had a key. Pam and Mike came to my apartment because they hadn't heard from me. They discovered me collapsed on the floor. They immediately dialed 911. I was taken to the emergency room at a hospital only four blocks away.

What happened in the emergency room?

They evaluated my condition. It was as if I was floating in the air, looking down at the doctors treating me. I'm not a particularly religious person. However, I saw myself and had a near-death experience. I was going in and out of consciousness, and I saw two angels and a wonderful light. [The] light was spectacular! I thought, "I want to go home to heaven. Send me home!" The two angels said, "You have a purpose here on earth. Not your time." And then I woke up in bed. I now know heaven exists.

How did you communicate?

I couldn't speak a word for more than two weeks after my stroke. I tried gestures, but they were difficult to do because my hands and legs were paralyzed. I was in a lot of pain, especially on my right side. I was in a wheelchair, so I communicated through blinking. One blink for yes, two blinks for no. Then came the red-letter day when I said my first word. I had a fruit basket in the day room, and my father pointed to an apple and asked, "What is it?" I said, "Apple." My dad started crying, and then my mom entered the room and also cried. It was about eighteen days after my stroke. I was very excited!

Did you go home after you left the rehab center?

I didn't go back to my apartment in San Francisco. I moved to El Dorado Hills, outside of Sacramento, California, where my parents live. I had speech therapy, occupational therapy, and physical therapy. After that, I had therapy at home. I kept going with a brace and a cane. My family helped me immensely. I believe that it takes a village to recover from a stroke.

For six years after my stroke, I was not able to say what I think; I was in a fog. I [still] get tired. I'm an intelligent person, but my mind gets overtired.

What do you miss most since your stroke?

Before my stroke, I had an active social life, but after the stroke, it stopped. I was depressed after I had the stroke. I was divorced several years before my stroke; I didn't have a husband or partner. I lost a lot of my friends from the San Francisco scene. Now I mostly rely on my family for support.

I have an active travel schedule because my family takes me on all sorts of trips: concerts in Las Vegas, Hawaii, cruises to Alaska, and so on. I am not able to read books, but I am able to comprehend my audio books. They are a godsend. My most challenging thing after the stroke was to be patient. I'm not in a hurry anymore. I had to slow down. I'm mellow. I think I'm intuitive. And I like that I've become intuitive.

What are your plans?

I want [to] learn something every day. I have a tutor, and I'm learning everything! Geography, etc. I'm recovering piece by piece. I'm empowering myself.

I continue to love taking trips on cruise ships, mostly to Hawaii. I dream of taking a trip around the world on a cruise ship. Before my stroke, I traveled to Bali three times. So I have never lost the travel bug.

As a stroke survivor, what do you recommend for family members and caregivers?
Be positive; be patient!

Commentary

Barb's stroke involved a thrombosis or blockage of the left proximal internal carotid artery, resulting in a large left middle cerebral artery infarct. This is the critical area for language. She had a history of hypertension, and her severe headaches were a warning of her impeding stroke.

Barb has gone from living the high life in the Financial District of San Francisco at forty-three years to her poststroke life in El Dorado Hills with her family to support her. She never lost her sparkle.

Every Wednesday, I see Barb sporting a cane and a big smile. Barb has an incredible vocabulary. She complains of having trouble with small words like articles and prepositions. After her stroke, Barb began recovering from Broca's aphasia. This form of aphasia is primarily an expressive problem. She can understand most everything that is said to her but has greater problems producing speech that matches her thoughts. Barb often points to her brain and says, "I have it here." Then she points to her mouth and says, "But it doesn't come out here." Her speech is telegraphic, and often she says the same thing she has said many times before. For example, in response to a question about her weekend or a trip she just took, she'll respond, "Had a good time." The depth of her thinking is far greater than she can express in words now. However, in almost every group session, she will give a surprisingly satisfying response that gratifies her and all of us in the group. She will say one word that is the perfect description of what the group is trying to say. For instance, when we are listing exotic fruits, she'll say, "Papaya." And then there is applause all around!

Today

Barb lives independently and is moving to a senior-living facility near her brother and sister. She has opted not to pursue driving and instead hires drivers to take her to group, movies, and shopping. She continues to travel and read audio books. She is at peace with her new lifestyle.

Barb in Bali Prestroke—Fearless!

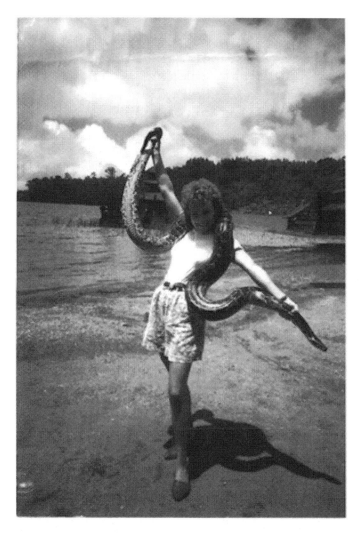

Pat, Barb's Mother

Tell me about your daughter's stroke.
Barb was living and working in San Francisco. It was on New Year's Eve. I got an e-mail from Barb saying she was going to go out that night and maybe to her sister Pam's the next day. The next day, New Year's Day, Pam called me, saying she was trying to get hold of Barb but couldn't. I told Pam that Barb was forty-four years old and had her own friends, but we didn't really know their phone numbers or where they lived. We didn't think any more of it.

Pam decided she would to go check on her sister. That's when Pam found her on the floor, barely breathing.

We heard about it, so of course we went to San Francisco right away. When we arrived, they told us she had a stroke. We didn't know the prognosis at that time. My husband and I moved into Barb's apartment in San Francisco right away. We stayed there for the whole time to be with her. She was in intensive care for a couple of days. Then she was moved to the rehabilitation unit in San Francisco.

What were your thoughts when you were heading to see her?
On our way, we were praying we would see her alive. We both thought, "Barb is young. Why her? Why not us?" Then, when we were told she might not walk again or speak, we were just devastated; we were heartbroken. However, we never gave up hope, because we knew she was a strong person and we are a strong family. I knew her brother and sister would back us up. We knew that if we could get her some help, she would be OK. We knew she couldn't go back to work. We just wanted her to live life and enjoy it, and she has certainly has.

Did you see any precursors of a stroke?
She did tell us before she had the stroke that she had migraines. At the financial business where she worked, they had a lot of televisions, and she told me they were giving her headaches. She did have high blood pressure, but she was taking medication for high blood pressure and was seeing a doctor for the headaches.

How was your experience at the hospital?

Well, the first six days was when she was in critical care. The doctor in charge was a specialist, not our family physician. He was very frank about what Barb had experienced and the way it was going to be. That was rather difficult because we were looking for a more positive outlook. However, the staff and the nurses were very sweet to us. Also, when they moved us to the rehab hospital, they were absolutely wonderful. We stayed at her apartment, so every day we would go to her early in the morning, and we would stay with her until night.

At the beginning, they were talking to us about a device that would help her talk with us. One of the most remarkable things was two weeks into her rehab, her father lifted up an apple and asked her what it was, and Barb said, "Apple." That was one of her first words since her stroke. We were just so thrilled. We knew she was going to get better.

Her sister and her brother would go and visit her for a day or two just to give us a little rest. Her little nieces went and supported her.

One of her best visitors was a gentleman who was a taxi driver. He had picked her up every morning while she was working. He just wanted to tell us how wonderful she was. It was just wonderful to hear the impact she had on people. She is my hero.

Did her personality change after the stroke?

She has never been shy about the stroke. For example, when we went to restaurants and I wanted to help her order because she had trouble ordering, I would tell her to take her time. It was hard—as a mom, you want to make everything right—but she had to learn how to do it herself. When she was more comfortable saying words like "hamburger," one of the things she started to say—not for pity, just to explain—was "I had a stroke." You would have been amazed at how people treated her. They would say "I'm sorry" and tell her to take her time. She is so open; she wants to help people understand she needs to take her time.

She loves the group because she gets to be with other people that have had a stroke and share the same experience. She is always learning. She comes home and tells me she was a star in reading.

She is more outgoing and loves to put herself out there. She also loves children. Before, she loved them, but now she even goes out of her way to talk to and spend time with them. She also has a real understanding of all types of people, not just people with disabilities.

Did your relationship change?
Before her stroke she focused on her career and business. Barb had her life in San Francisco. We would see her once a month and talk to her on the phone.

After the stroke, she lived with us for about a year. We take care of her finances and bills. Now she lives in her own apartment a mile from us, and someone comes three times a week to take her to group or to a movie. She comes to eat throughout the week, and we also take her out to eat since she loves eating. I do a lot of shopping with her and also make her appointments. She is independent because I can't do everything with her, but I certainly go to all her doctor appointments. She goes in and knows what the doctor tells her, but it is harder for her to tell us what the doctor told her, so it is easier to go with her.

How do you think Barb feels about her stroke?
She went through some very tough times. She went from having a lot of friends and traveling to many places by herself to now traveling with family. She has learned to accept it.

She knows she can improve her speech and reading. She reads, but it gets tiring. So we found audio books. She always has ten or thirteen books in her MP3 player. She listens to her books three to four hours a day. Having had a stroke doesn't stop her from doing many of the things she did before; she goes to plays and travels.

What has been the biggest challenge going through this journey with Barb?
[Barb] has a new way of life. [She is] not who she [once] was. She is still fearless, of course, but she can't drive. If she wants to go somewhere or do something, she has to ask. For example, if she runs out of milk, she has to call. That

[asking for help] is a big challenge for her. And one of our challenges was to accept the new Barb.

Another thing was not to over mother her but to allow her to grow and have her own opinions. Even when I was worried sometimes, I would let her be her, because, after all, she is fifty-five. She is old enough and aware enough to make her own decisions. Even when they are at that age, you want to do everything right for them, but you have to let them be themselves. That is why we wanted to get someone from the agency (Visiting Angels, senior-care services) so if she wanted to go to the movies and we couldn't, she would still be able to go.

How is Barb in public?
In public, even when she doesn't know someone, she will say, "Hi, I'm Barb," and will not be shy about telling people she had a stroke. She is the same person. We know other people who have had a stroke and withdrawn. You can't believe the things she does. When we were on a cruise, she would stay after dinner, listening to music. She would go to the piano bar, and we would go back to our room. The next morning people would tell her, "Hey, Barb, didn't we have fun at the bar last night?" She is very outgoing and friendly.

What would be your advice to other parents in the same situation as yours?
You have to have a positive attitude and a heart full of love for your child and what he or she is going through. Also a sense of hope, because the medical personnel will tell you that this and that won't come back. You have to have hope so you have a positive attitude. I never told her she would never be able to drive again or travel to Europe by herself, but we have always given her hope that we would make it happen with her nieces and siblings. You have to have hope because there are many advances in research and medicine. My husband was a colonel in the air force, and we see all these young men who have been injured, but we always see them living a full life. There is always a tomorrow. We also give Barb something to look forward to. For example, we tell her we will go to a play, go on a cruise, or go see her sister. We always try to be on the same page.

Commentary

Everyone who has had a stroke, especially with aphasia, needs an advocate. Being helpful but allowing for independence is challenging, especially for parents of an adult child who has had a stroke. Another parent—Jason's father, Bob, in chapter 5—also had to face this dilemma.

Eight

The Chess Master: The Doctor Had Three Strokes, but He's Not Out!

*D*on is our longest attendee in the Sentence Structure Group. He has had three strokes, his first one at age fifty. He carries a cane, walks erect, and is tall for a short man. His physique betrays his passion for soccer, which he played for most of his life. His second passion is chess, and although he has Broca's aphasia, his language deficits have not affected his play of the game. Chess is a nonverbal logical and strategic game; both these skills are undiminished by Don's strokes. He plays four or five games on a computer simultaneously. His PhD was in criminal justice, and by his own admission, he was a hard-ass gun-toting guy. He is now happy to play chess and garden, and he religiously comes to group. When asked about his strokes, he responds without a bit of irony, "Oh well, I'm not dead yet."

Here is Don's story.

Tell us about your strokes.
I was teaching at the university in Sacramento when I had my first stroke. Before moving to Sacramento, I was a police detective in Dallas, where I got my PhD. My wife, Linda, and I have three children, all girls. One of our

daughters recently completed her degree in speech pathology. I think she was motivated to go into speech pathology because of my stroke.

I had three strokes. The first one was in 2005, the second one in 2006, and the third 2010. When the first one happened, I told my wife, "Linda, I feel bad, but I'm going to work anyway." The next morning my wife said, "Let's go see the doctor." I didn't think about a stroke; I just felt bad.

We went to Mercy Hospital in Elk Grove, California, where the doctors diagnosed my stroke. The doctors kept me in the hospital for three days so they could monitor my progress. After that, they gave me medications and told me to go home. I didn't feel that I had many effects from that stroke.

You had three strokes in total, and yet you survived!
Then the second one was in 2006, and I thought I was going to die! I consider myself a really tough guy. I don't give up easily. I was [a] police detective in Dallas, after all. But it just hit me like a ton of bricks.

I tried to call 911, but my muscles were numb. I couldn't talk. I couldn't do anything. I thought, "I am fifty-three years old, and I've had another stroke, and I'm going to die." Mercy Hospital put me in intensive care, but I don't remember much about my time in intensive care.

After the first three weeks [I] was in intensive care, I thought, "I am going to be OK." About six months later, I went to rehab for speech therapy and physical therapy. I went to UCDMC for speech therapy, and I went to a local community college for physical therapy. Then I enrolled in the Sacramento State program, which teaches young students how to be speech therapists. I am there as a great example for them, what they have to face while working in the profession and how to deal with people with stroke outcomes like mine.

The third stroke happened in 2010. I thought, "Not again!" That stroke happened when my father was dying. I loved him a great deal, and I think I had a stroke because he was dying. He lived in Virginia, and I lived in Sacramento, so we were far apart in distance but close in our relationship. I was in the hospital for three weeks and finally said, "I'm going to see my dad." I couldn't stay in rehab during that time, and fortunately, I got to see Dad before he died.

What was the biggest challenge after your strokes?

I can't use my right hand, and my right leg is impaired; I have to use a cane and am fortunate not to be in a wheelchair. I can't use my right hand to write, but I can talk pretty well. I cannot drive, but I can use Para transportation. I still think really well, and I like to play chess. I'm even pretty good at it. Not as good as I was before my stroke, but I hold my own! All in all, my thinking is great, but I just can't get my thoughts from my brain to my mouth.

What are the lessons you learned after your stroke?

I have learned to be closer to my wife. We've been married for forty years, and she just rolls with the punches. I think [my] having strokes made our marriage stronger. Before my strokes, I was a big, fierce guy, and I was mad all the time. Now, I am very peaceful. I am at peace with myself and everybody else.

Initially, I was depressed after each of my strokes. About five years ago, I was kind of depressed. I thought I was going to learn to read and write, but I can't yet. I'm going to pull through this. I am a fighter, and that's what I'm going to do.

What advice do you have for the medical professionals who took care of you?

Talking to them was difficult. They couldn't understand me, and I couldn't understand them. They talked so fast, and they talked all at once.

What do you enjoy now?

I am very active. I enjoy the college students at Sacramento State; I go there at least twice a week. I go to the Sentence Structure Group at University of California Davis Medical Center [once] a week also. But what I really enjoy is playing chess and working in my garden.

Commentary

Don has moderate to severe Broca's aphasia. He also has alexia[21] and agraphia.[22] He is almost entirely unable to read. He can, however, read numbers and

---

21 Alexia is the inability to read.
22 Agraphia is the inability to write.

do calculations. He has great difficulty finding the word he is trying to say. Given time and an initial sound cue, Don can often say the target word. He is emphatic that the word he is trying to say is often in his head, but not always. Don says, "Having the stroke was wonderful; it completely changed me. My wife and I are really happy, and that is after thirty-nine years." His wife, Linda, completely agrees.

Today

Don attends our group and another support group weekly. He also goes to the university speech-therapy program and participates in their classes three days a week. He is constantly working to maintain his independence and language skills. He recently received a state award from the California Speech-Language-Hearing Association for being a positive role model for individuals with aphasia. Because he does not drive, he uses Paratransit to attend all his activities. He continues to play chess and garden.

Linda, Don's Wife

Tell me about Don's strokes. He has had three over the past five years.
The first stroke was extremely mild. He went right back to work. He just had some numbness and recovered almost 100 percent. At that point the doctors did not prescribe anything, since the first stroke was so mild. Then he had a seizure while shopping in 2006, and we went straight to the hospital. It was with his second stroke in 2006 that he acquired aphasia. That one was the one that opened our eyes as to what the effects of a stroke were. He was on leave from work for a year, and eventually, he knew he was not going to be able to go back to work.

Did he have any therapies?
He went to rehabilitation for a week, and they released him home because he could get around. We decided to take him to physical and speech therapy versus home therapy because he was able to walk, but very slowly. He didn't have the cane at that point.

How did his personality change after the stroke?
On the second stroke, he was extremely angry. He was upset, and it affected all of us. It affected my youngest the most, as she was not able to grasp what had happened to the daddy she knew. She couldn't understand it at all. She was Daddy's baby, so it was very hard for her. I wasn't sure how bad it was going to get. He wanted to go back to work. There was a lot to think about. He was very determined and adamant about what he could do himself. I tried to calm him, but he was very scared; we all were.

How did his personality change after his third stroke?
He was more resigned and said, "Here we go again." He was past the anger. When the third stroke happened, he thought he would have to start all over. He was unhappy, but he knew he had done it before and he could do it again. He was not going to give up.

At what point did he make that turn where he was not so angry anymore?

It was a year after the second stroke. He started therapy at the Sacramento State speech-therapy department. He went through three therapists because he was so angry. It was the saddest thing; we had to apologize for him. They worked with him, and after he realized he was getting better and started talking, he liked it more and more, and his attitude started to change because he saw the improvement he was making. He began to love going to those sessions because he wanted to get better and better. We also worked with him at home.

How did your youngest daughter feel?

When it first happened, she had to move out and stay with my older daughter because she felt she had to get away from the stress at home. She never stopped loving him, obviously. She called him all the time, even when she was out of town. But she was very young, only nineteen. This transition was huge for our family, and the way he responded to her hurt her feelings. She did not know what to do and was totally lost and upset.

I want to hear your perspective.

My mother was staying with us, so that allowed me to go back to work. Otherwise, I would've had to quit. She was elderly and very opinionated. She and Don sometimes tangled a bit.

It was a confusing time for me, and I blanked out a lot of it because it was such an ordeal. I didn't know anyone who had had a stroke, and I had nothing to go by. I had to Google my questions and search for information constantly. We owned our house, and I even decided at that point I needed to sell the house. I just didn't know whether we were going to go on living here, because all our family was back in Texas.

We eventually put our house up for sale. I was trying to make plan A and plan B scenarios. It was a lot, and no one could really help me with those decisions. There are just a lot of things you have to think about. You first have to make sure your family is stable.

How did you survive this?

I had to shift to a different mind-set. I had to think, "What needs to be done?" I was very fortunate to have family members to help me. At the same time, I had to work with Don. It was especially hard because I was trying to help him more than he wanted to help himself. I kept reading, and I was constantly on the lookout to see what I could do. When I found organizations that might help, I would contact them. I reached out to the resources I found online. He had not worked long enough at the university to have insurance coverage, and he didn't have retirement savings to fall back on either. It fell to me to feed our family, so I simply had to keep working. We eventually sold the house and struggled with the emotions of it. I was just so focused. I was determined that we weren't going to lose everything.

Don started his therapy, and he started to develop into a more positive person. That helped me a lot. He was independent enough that I could arrange his transportation. I learned about Paratransit. Don was not able to board the bus by himself, so I had to work with the bus company for those arrangements too. It was just so much that I felt on the verge of being drained most of the time. Luckily, I had a lot of energy, because he needed me to have a lot of energy. But I also needed to let him do as much as he could for himself. I tried to push him so he would start to do more and more for himself.

We wanted Don to get better enough to go back to work, but we sat down and talked about him resigning his position at the university. They were holding his job for him, but I couldn't imagine him standing in front of a class and talking. His speech has never improved enough to teach.

I could not have done it without all the help I got, especially my mother's help. I needed someone I trusted to talk to.

Don now has acquired all these phrases of encouragement: "You need to move on" and "Keep going." Now he encourages not only people who have had a stroke but everyone.

Your life has changed a lot.

Yes, I have to do pretty much everything now. He used to pay the bills, so after his strokes I had to learn how to deal with all the financial stuff. My oldest daughter was already in the speech-pathology program at the university, so her assistance helped our predicament immensely. I also had my friends and my manager at work who supported me.

What do you do to take care of yourself?
After all these years, my daughter and I finally joined a gym. I like to read as I give myself some "me time." My mother and I did some mini shopping trips, and I also picked up crocheting when I found it was very relaxing. I just felt the need to clear my mind. Sometimes I'd go in the backyard and just drink some wine.

How were you sleeping?
I was not sleeping very well at the beginning, but then when Don was relaxing and happier, I started to sleep better and have fewer worries. We have created a routine now: watch our favorite shows and then relax in the yard for a while. It is more relaxing, and we get along very well with this routine. When he is happy, I am happy.

I had to do everything at the very beginning, but now he comforts me. He even gets me a glass of wine in the evening. Comforting each other is where we are at right now.

Do you have any other advice for people?
I truly believe you have to know the personality of your loved one. For Don, I had to learn to let him do what he wanted to do, and I always tried to keep him busy. I pushed him to his limit so he could start to be independent and do whatever he wanted for himself.

Encourage them to be as independent as they can be, and encourage them do things for themselves. This gives them the opportunity to work and stay engaged. I did what I was comfortable with and helped him while at the same time letting him be as independent as possible. He likes that I am always checking on him, and he is OK with my loving concern.

The Chess Master's Number-Three Daughter

What was your relationship like with your father?
I was close to my father. He was the go-to person for everything, even boy-friends if I got in trouble. I used to run to my father, not my mom. We had an amazing relationship.

His first stroke happened when I was eighteen. I didn't understand any-thing about a stroke. His right arm was affected, and he was a little standoffish.

What happened after his second stroke?
His second stroke changed everything. I was at work, and my mom called and asked me to come home: "It's about Daddy." Mom and my sisters were all affected by his inability to speak. He was frustrated and angry and could be mean to us. He said things he didn't mean to say, and sometimes it wasn't what he said but how he said it. He couldn't say our names. We were daughters number one, two, and three. I was number three. At dinner he would sit with his eyes closed tightly because he was so overwhelmed by the confusion caused by our conversation.

Did therapy help?
We were told by the speech therapist to talk slower, a lot slower, but it was still a guessing game to understand what he wanted. He would say a word, "the dog," but it was way off target from what he wanted to say. We would argue because I was not able to guess what he was trying to say, so I'd walk away. It could take fifteen minutes for him to get one sentence out. It was very dif-ficult, and I ultimately steered clear of him.

How did your relationship change?
I drove him to his speech class. He would cuss and say words like "shit" and "dick" that he didn't mean, or he would lash out at someone. It was embar-rassing for us. His reactions really embarrassed me. I always had to step in and

explain to others what he meant. I also had to stand up for him. It was a role reversal, and I had to be in charge of him.

He also didn't seem to want anything to do with us. He was confused. It was tough because I was pregnant at that time. Paradoxically, I was also angry and frustrated, so my feelings were similar to his.

My dad was an extremely intelligent man, a professor, and a soccer referee. I felt so bad for him when I could say what he couldn't. Day to day he must have wondered whether he was going to get well enough to teach again.

How is your relationship now?
He has become more peaceful now. The big change in roles has been with my mom. My mother is selfless. After seeing her in action, I realize she is the rock. She would give you the shirt off her back. She is the strongest and most patient person I know.

Nine

MIKE: AN ENGINEER'S APPROACH TO STROKE RECOVERY

Mike is an engineer. He worked for HP at the time of his stroke at age forty-eight. He is the father of two; his son, Alex, has graduated, and his youngest, Nichole, is in college. His wife, Victoria, is a psychologist in private practice.

Mike is determined to regain much of his capability but has found speech therapy frustrating. He attended group and participated in research briefly. Victoria has always managed the social calendar and continues to do so. As a result, Mike has maintained many of his close friendships. They camp and dine together. This is rare and speaks highly of Mike's personality and the commitment of his friends.

This is Mike's story.

What were you feeling when you were having a stroke?
[Mike points to his wife.] I don't remember. I do, but I don't remember what I was feeling. It is in the morning when I got to the ER. At p.m. I was talking, and they gave me the medicine. Then I couldn't talk. The tPA cleaned it up, some of it; it got loose and blocked the carotid artery.

What symptoms did you have?
I don't think I had headaches. Well, I don't remember. [Mike points to his wife.] I was in the hospital for two days, and then I woke up, and I couldn't talk.

What happened after the stroke?

I don't remember the first words I said. I just remember thinking, "I am getting better." I would say maybe little by little. Everything was lost. I didn't know what I was looking at. I was at the hospital for a month. I can't remember if I had speech. I was here at UC Davis Medical Center.

What are some of the things you work on?

I have been getting better. I have been doing Rosetta Stone for the past two weeks ago. I work on pronouns, and the little words are the worst.

What are some of the problems you face?

I have trouble talking on the phone. With Rosetta, I say it, not just think it! I am better at solving problems. I know a lot about physics.

Did you keep your close friendships?

I have kept a lot of my friends from HP, Sineal, Chris, and Ed, a little bit less here and there. I've known them for a long time. Just this past weekend, I cooked for them. We chatted a little, and I made the cooking. The level of talking is lower, and I can keep up. My friends are from long time ago. We watched videos of going to Yosemite. We are all going camping next week.

Tell me about your family.

I have Alex, my son; he went somewhere close to a place. The place's name has five to six letters in it. My son got his degree in computers and works in video games. I also have a daughter, Nichole, who is the youngest and is now studying English and French.

How have your children adjusted to your stroke?

I don't know. It has been a hard time. Nichole had a problem at the end of high school.

How much has your personality changed?
[Mike shrugs, and his wife responds.] He has always been very humble and modest. He does not show much of himself. He is very self-confident and has high standards for himself.

Commentary

Mike's brain scan shows extensive damage to the language system in the left hemisphere. Mike exhibits both expressive language problems and comprehension problems. It is very difficult for him to express himself thoroughly unless it is to someone who knows him very well, like his wife.

Mike's Brain Scan[23]

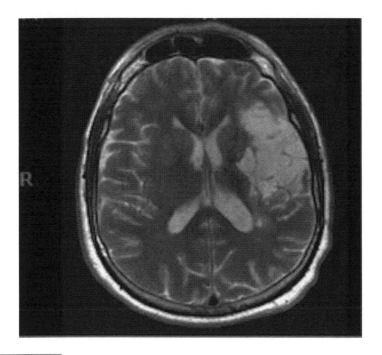

_____

23 Scan orientation: the right side of the MRI correlates with the left brain and the left with the right. The white area shows a large left middle cerebral artery infarct due to a carotid artery dissection. This caused a blockage in the artery that feeds blood and oxygen to the left hemisphere.

Victoria, Mike's Wife

Tell me about the stroke.

Mike's stroke was April 9, 2013. Looking back, we realize there were stroke symptoms we didn't notice. The night before the stroke, Mike said to me, "I have had this headache for the past two days." We didn't know they were stroke symptoms at the time. His vision was blurry as well. I said this didn't sound good. I had just read an article about stroke symptoms. The article was about a man who was cooking and dropped dead. I told Mike about that and said, "You know this doesn't sound good. Shouldn't you go in?" He dismissed it, of course; you know how guys are. When something hurts, I immediately start complaining, but Mike doesn't complain.

It was not until the middle of the night, around three o'clock, that he woke up, and he was holding his hand up and trying to wake me up. He has a really high pain tolerance. He was just staring at me; I realized he was trying to move his right hand. He wanted to tell me he couldn't move his right hand. So I knew he was having a stroke.

What were you feeling?

[Mike answers.] Nothing. I didn't feel anything.

Do you have any family history of stroke?

His grandmother on his dad's side had a stroke in her early fifties. She lived to be in her seventies; she was cared for by her younger daughter. His great-grandmother had a stroke at forty-nine and died. We found this out later. This is something we didn't know.

Did he have any health problems before the stroke?

He had high blood pressure. He had taken a statin, and it was controlled. He saw his primary physician before the stroke. His cholesterol was getting high.

What happened after you noticed he was having a stroke?

I called my daughter, Nichole. She was in her last year of high school. I told her to stay with her dad because I was trying to call 911. We lived out in the country, but they came fairly quickly. They came in probably ten or fifteen minutes. I told them what was happening, and I asked them whether this was a stroke.

They said, "I can't tell you." They put an oxygen mask on him, and he started talking. I thought maybe it was an oxygen thing, but it just happened to clear up a little bit. He could walk and talk a little bit. They took him in the ambulance, and Nichole and I drove to the hospital. He got admitted to the ER right way. When we got there, he was talking pretty normally. They did physical and cognitive tests. Then they did some scans and said something had happened. We were waiting, and I was sitting there thinking I needed to cancel the appointments I had scheduled for the next day. So I was doing some of that, but he was speaking pretty normally. Then a lot of the doctors left the room, and I asked Mike whether he had told the doctor he had had an aspirin. I asked him three times the same question; that was when I realized something was wrong.

So I called for the doctor, and I told them he was not answering me. They were not sure it was a stroke. It was later when we found out the headache and the blindness in his eye were related to the stroke.

Then they asked whether we would like to try tPA and explained it all. They tested something else to make sure it was OK to give him tPA. We were there while they injected the tPA in the ER. He was doing well; he was naming a lot of pictures. Then things started to get worse. He didn't notice, but we did. We have some videos of him talking at that time.

Then what happened?
They said he seemed to be responding and they were going to put him in the neuro ICU. He was in the ICU for eight days, and because our insurance is through UC Davis, they transferred him to UC Davis ICU. He spent about five days in the ICU there. He then went to the rehabilitation unit. He had a feeding tube placed. His swallowing was fine; it was just a precaution. So the hospital stay was a total of a month and a half.

How was your stay at the hospital?
They were all very nice, but I wanted to be there all the time. Nichole would come and stay for a little bit. His father came and my brother came. His

friends came, but I knew he would not want his friends to see him in his robe. Nobody saw him then, only his father and my brother. I told his friends not to visit, because I didn't want to put that on him. There was plenty of time for friends to come and visit after he was home. They respected that, but what they did—and this is very wonderful—is they started this Google web group. He worked at HP, and he was a manager for a long time. Everybody loved him. We would write down on the website what was going on. There were about eighty people following the website.

My book club also did something great: they started a meal plan. The HP family and the book club collaborated to do the meal plan. His friends took care of me. It was nice because that way I didn't have to worry about what to cook or about Nichole. It was nice that people helped. When he was out of the hospital, they were able to continue the meals and visit him. He was able to see his friends. I asked them to keep it short. It was nice.

Going back to that first day at the hospital, his friend Jon came to visit, and he sat down with me to talk. Jon filtered what was happening to the HP group. Probably the next day, his boss, Ed, came over with Brian and Sunil; they are the four musketeers. Ed thinks of Brian, Sunil, and Mike as his sons. They think of one another as brothers. Mike has a real brother, but he has never come by. So I am glad we have friends.

How did you feel during this ordeal?
I don't think I was scared. Because I am a therapist, I have been trained to observe. I was kind of observing myself, and I was strangely calm. I look back to calling 911 and getting through everything we needed to take care of. There were times when he stopped responding; I had to call the nurse and make them do something. They would tell me this was normal, but I would tell them I didn't want him to go into a coma or to have something happen to him.

That is the thing, backtracking a little bit. He was in the ICU on April 9 in the afternoon, five or six o'clock. Nichole went to school a half day, and Mike kept telling me to go home because Nichole needed me. I noticed when they came in to do the cognitive test that he wasn't doing better; he was getting worse. So I asked the nurse, "Why is he getting worse? Can you call the doctor and ask? Because I don't feel this is right." I went home for just a couple of hours. I called the hospital, and the doctor told me he would wax and wane, but I told him I was seeing him only waning.

We went back, Nichole and I; it was probably nine o'clock. We went in there, and he wasn't talking or moving his right side. There was a full pee jar, and the nurse said it must have been thirty minutes since he had used it. What they told us later is they did a scan and an ultrasound and there was an arterial dissection on the left side. They said nobody would do surgery because it was too dangerous. It is better to have a blockage and have a stroke. It was a major carotid artery. It was the tissue inside his artery, and his cholesterol didn't help. Things had started to collect inside his artery. When the tPA started to work, it pulled off a little plaque, which moved a little higher and blocked the artery. So he actually had the full stroke there in the hospital, and we couldn't do anything about it. This was when I was gone for two hours. It was even happening there in the hospital, with all the waiting and waiting. The tPA could have contributed [to the damage]; however, it could have been worse and affected more. I don't know how far it went up, but it broke off a piece [of plaque]. Mike often has asked me about it, and I tell him about it each time.

The thing about that morning of April 9 is he was supposed to go with his friend Kevin to a conference. It was some kind of tech conference, and he was going to drive. It was great he didn't go.

Commentary

Victoria, like Kathleen (chapter 4), wonders what she could have done differently in the initial moments of her spouse's stroke. Both she and Kathleen are devoted wives and highly educated; going forward, they feel they have a sense of responsibility to others like themselves. Their stories are an effort to inform wives and husbands about the challenges of being the spouse of a stroke survivor.

A few months ago, Mike and his wife read about some research Stanford was doing. They were injecting stem cells into the brains of stroke survivors to improve outcome. Mike was adamant about pursuing inclusion in this study. They contacted Sambio Co., which was collaborating with UCSF and Stanford, and underwent prescreening. They sent off his MRI scans and medical records. Unfortunately, the researchers determined that the area of damage was too large and Mike did not meet the criteria for inclusion.

Today

Mike has not returned to work. He mentions that he misses the people at work. However, he is constantly working at home. He has been learning to program a Raspberry Pi[24] by watching instructions on YouTube. He continues to enjoy programming, but once he gets stuck, even his HP friends admit that helping him is beyond them because Mike's computer skills are so advanced.

A year and a half ago, he took the written test to get his driver's license back. He had his car modified so he can use his left leg for the brake and accelerator. He also has a knob on the steering wheel to help him steer with his left hand. He passed both the written and driving tests and consequently has gained more independence.

He can do routine errands such as going to the post office or grocery store, driving to his therapy at the hospital outpatient clinic, and driving his wife to work. He orders from restaurants he is very familiar with, such as Quiznos and Togo's. Victoria tells a story about when they were going to meet for lunch in separate cars and she got lost. Mike called her on her cell phone because he was worried about where she was. She laughs; it is usually Victoria that is worried about Mike!

Victoria says they have always been very close, although independent. Even now they are in sync. She says, "Even now Mike can still finish my sentences."

Mike does Rosetta Stone for English and attends speech therapy once a week. More than anything he wants to read orally. For fifteen to twenty minutes a day, Victoria reads as Mike follows along. Mike feels he is getting better,

---

24 Raspberry Pi is a tiny and affordable computer that you can use to learn programming through fun, practical projects.

"little by little." He is going back to occupational therapy for his arm and gets Botox every two months to address the tone. His social life remains as it was before his stroke, in large part because he is so highly regarded by his friends and colleagues and because of his wife's commitment to keeping their friends in their lives. Mike seems happier and more relaxed these days.

Victoria and Mike are planning a trip to France this summer, and Victoria has returned to her private practice as a psychologist.

Ten

BECKY: PARTY ON TO RECOVERY!

*B*ecky is a beloved third-grade teacher. She received her master's degree from the University of the Pacific (UOP). She earned the Teacher of the Year award two years before her stroke. She has close ties with the local music community. She loves socializing: music, singing, dancing, and hanging with her friends. Before her stroke Becky volunteered to be the surrogate mother for a couple who otherwise could not have children. These were musician friends of hers, and she has remained close to them.

Becky had her stroke at age forty-four. Since she has regained mobility and language skills, she has flirted with the idea of rehabilitating dogs, particularly pit bulls. She was inspired by a documentary she saw about the rehabilitation of pit bulls abused as fighting dogs. She feels she can do this type of work with her limited language skills and it will provide meaning to her life. She is passionate about this.

Here is her story.

Tell us how your stroke occurred.
I was having dinner with friends at Christmastime, December 27, 2014. I had a headache, a real bad headache. I didn't know; I had no idea then. I had

a seizure in front of all my friends. One was a veterinarian, and she took my vitals. They called 911. I really don't remember anything after that.

What is the first thing you remember?
The first thing I remember was walking with a nurse and playing cards. I was in a group, and there was a man and woman talking in Spanish. I was having trouble talking, and it confused me. I was in a wheelchair, and Katy, my wife, was there.

I remember all my friends came and played music at the hospital. They played the guitar and sang in the therapy room. They rolled me in, and there was Chris, Kathy, and Tracy. There were stuffed animals and cards. All my friends came and brought sandwiches and drinks and hung out in my hospital room.

Did you have therapy?
I remember the occupational therapist said my right arm was "dead." Physical therapy took me on the parallel bars. In outpatient I saw Kyle [speech therapist]; he is a hella funny guy. Also went to group on Fridays with seven other people.

Do you have any advice?
Get better, talking, walking in the trees and flowers. Take time to smell the roses. Work, work, then sleep. I enjoy watching Netflix and playing music. I'm smelling the roses; before, I was too busy.

Family and friends should slow down, speak slow. Ask questions, like Don in our group asks, "How are you?" Go out to lunch with all the guys. Hang out.

What is the most important thing to you now?
The most important thing is friends, family, people, love, playing cards, playing games, music, backgammon, and movies. Get better. I am a stroke survivor, and I'm getting stronger.

Commentary

Becky has Broca's aphasia and has great difficulty inserting verbs into her sentences. She has a fantastic support team: her wife, Katy; her two brothers; musician friends; her dad in Iowa; and her mom in Washington. The Sentence Structure Group has met all these people because they have asked permission to observe the group so they know how to help her. She has good days and bad. Some days she says one sentence after another. Roz, her friend and caretaker, helps her communicate and plays cognitive games with her. Roz is pretty amazing; she is patient, talks slowly, and waits for Becky to get her thoughts out, helping only when necessary. So many friends and family being devoted to Becky is a testament to the person she is.

Today

Becky is more independent than ever, but she does not drive. She is mobile with a slight right hemiparesis of her arm and leg. She has not returned to work. Her close friend Roz provides transportation and companionship. She often flies up to visit her mom in Washington, and she stays in close contact with her dad.

Becky's brain scan shows more damage to the anterior aspect of the left hemisphere than the posterior. She has greater problems expressing herself than she does understanding what is said to her. Her oral reading and comprehension are superior to her expressive speech.

Becky's Brain Scan[25]

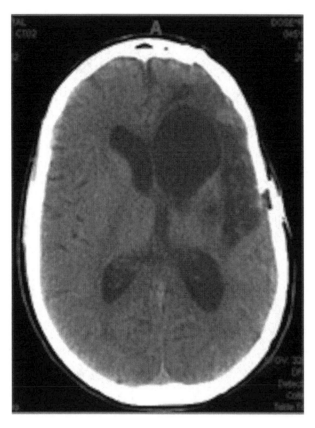

25 The CT scan shows results after the clipping of an internal carotid artery aneurysm. Minimal residual from a left-sided subarachnoid hemorrhage and right frontoparietal subdural fluid collection. Sequelae of prior left middle cerebral artery territory infarct, with encephalomalacia (softening or loss of brain tissue after cerebral infarction or other injury—the term is usually used to describe blurred cortical margins and decreased consistency of brain tissue after infarction) and ex vacuo dilatation of the left lateral ventricle, which is stable.

Becky's Mom: Don't Mess with Mama Bear

Becky had a brain aneurysm[26] on December 27, which was a Saturday night. Becky's mom learned about her stroke from her son that evening. She left her home in the state of Washington on the first flight to Sacramento, where Becky was in the intensive care unit at Kaiser Hospital.

You had to travel quite a distance; you must have been worried about Becky.
It was too late at night to catch a flight that evening from Seattle, so I had to wait till the morning to fly down to Sacramento. To put it simply, I was terrified! I was afraid Becky wouldn't survive the night. I was afraid I wouldn't get there in time. My son made my flight reservations. As the night unfolded, we got more details.

Once you arrived in Sacramento, what happened?
In the first couple of weeks, there was one procedure after another. She had a thirteen-hour craniotomy[27] (it also involved rerouting the blood flow in her brain by using a twelve-inch section of artery from her left arm), ventricular drain, and removal of a brain flap to reduce the brain swelling. I went from fearful to positive as she survived each procedure. Visitors were limited during her two-month hospitalization.

What did you do to take care of yourself?
I prayed a lot. There was a chapel at the hospital, so I went there to pray. Becky had been through so much, surviving two bouts of cancer in the past four years and now this! I prayed to God, "Why not take me? Why her?"

Midway through her hospitalization at Kaiser, there was pressure from Becky's insurance company and the office staff at Kaiser to transfer her to a general floor at UC Davis Medical Center (UCDMC). We felt this was premature, owing to her condition, and contacted her operating neurosurgeon. We learned he agreed with us and did not support the transfer! Several weeks later, when she was stable enough to be transferred, I helped her Kaiser

---

26 An aneurysm is an enlargement of an artery due to weakness in the artery wall.
27 A craniotomy is the surgical removal of a part of the skull.

neurosurgeon apply for temporary privileges at UCDMC so he could continue to follow her progress. (I knew about the credentialing process because I worked for thirty years in medical staff services as director.)

She was then transferred to UCDMC. Weeks later, her Kaiser neurosurgeon performed the bone-flap replacement at UCDMC. We were told the doctor personally carried the flap to the UCDMC, performed the surgery, and followed her progress. She needed me to advocate for her and question the decisions of the insurance company and office staff. No one was going to mess with Mama Bear!

Were you ever discouraged by her progress?
At one point early in her hospitalization, I had a hard time. The nurses had to restrain her from getting out of bed because she could not walk and she didn't understand the danger. She was fighting me, and she yelled and screamed at me when I would prevent her from getting up if the wheelchair was not near. That was devastating! A nurse said, "This is common. She's going to take her anger and frustration out on you because moms are safe." That actually made me feel better.

I loved her progress and determination! She'd try to smile and say hi to everybody she met. I thought, "She is going to make it. She'll keep trying." I had a succession of feelings: from fear about how much strength and speech she could regain to knowing she would overcome the obstacles, as she always had in the past. I loved being with her, and I cherished every moment with her. I was just thankful she was alive!

That must have been a difficult time. Were you afraid?
Initially, when I arrived at the hospital, the day after her stroke, I was very fearful; the prognosis was not good. I was having heart palpitations. My blood pressure was being monitored. If I have any advice, it's don't show the patient your fear. Think positive! During the initial stages of Becky's hospitalization, some people came into the room, saw Becky in her condition, and started crying. I quickly escorted them out of the room until they could compose themselves. Mama Bear says no negative energy allowed!

After Becky's release from the hospital, I wasn't sure how much she could remember from the past, so I showed her a photo album of her and her two brothers as children. I told her about all the happy times she had as a child. Then she began to remember the happy times of her childhood. Her brother came to visit from Germany twice, staying for two weeks each time. Her younger brother from Washington State also made two trips to Sacramento to be with her. Her father came from Iowa. Everyone—Katy, family, and friends—rallied around Becky.

In the hospital, we would rub her limbs and do exercises on her right side, as it was paralyzed. Physical therapy taught us to encourage movement on her right side. It was important to keep her moving all the time.

What therapies did she have?

She had occupational therapy, physical therapy, and speech therapy in the hospital at Kaiser and UCDMC. She got out of the hospital the last of February. We had to wait for the insurance to kick in for outpatient therapy. She received her therapies from Rehab Without Walls, which came to her home to provide services. Rehab Without Walls was great since Becky tired easily and the trips to outside facilities would tire her even more.

Has Becky changed since her stroke?

Initially she had trouble walking, and she can't see from her left eye. It's frustrating for her not to be able to speak as fluently as before the stroke.

She has always been a very loving, happy, giving person. But she now seems happier and more giving than before! We have always been close, Becky and I, but since her stroke, we are closer. I am more protective of her. I'm always watching out to see whether she's going to trip on something, such as a curb or sidewalk or dog.

She is thankful to be alive, and I am thankful also. One day, I was standing in the bathroom brushing my teeth; she stopped and observed me for a while, smiled, and said, "I love you, Mom." She doesn't feel sorry for herself. She is still connected to children; she buys books and clothes for children she knows, and she even made a video of bedtime stories. She's always commenting about the birds singing and flying overhead, smelling the flowers, and feeling the warmth of the sun.

Her stroke occurred at the end of December, during the school holiday break, so she didn't have a chance to say good-bye to her third-graders. She got cards and e-mails from her third-graders missing her and wishing her well. She recently went to see her third-grade class, now fourth-graders, to say good-bye and explain what happened to her. Even the boys cried and cried. She misses teaching the kids and her friends at school. However, she doesn't miss the constantly changing regulations involved with teaching.

What advice would you give family members?
Read all you can about your loved one's condition, loss of sight, aphasia, and stroke. In addition to a lot of online reading, I read *My Stroke of Insight* by Jill Bolte Taylor twice, and *The Art of Seeing with One Eye*. During Becky's two-month hospitalization, her wife, Katy, and I would take turns being with Becky twenty-four-seven. Becky always knew we were close by. We always offered love and encouragement, nothing negative. Don't let your loved one see you cry; be positive. Keep a stiff upper lip. Be a Mama Bear when the doctors and administrators try to push you around. Everybody needs an advocate. You are the patient's advocate.

Katy, Becky's Wife

How would you describe the circumstances surrounding Becky's stroke?
It was a complete shock. There were no signs it was going to happen. She was at a dinner party. Roz, our friend, had driven her to the party, and I was going to meet them later. She'd been gone for only about thirty minutes when the phone started buzzing. I looked at the text, and it said there was an emergency and to go to the hospital immediately. After I got there, things became a blur, so I don't remember many of the details. They had sedated and examined her and then told us what they were going to do. I was scared to death. The first information I got was that she wasn't going to make it. They said it was a miracle she made it to the emergency room. I honestly wanted to feel positive. Negative was not what I wanted to feel, but everything I was hearing was not good. I had a lot of thoughts, but mostly I was thinking, "What will I do without her?"

Tell us about your experience being with Becky at the hospital.
I was at the hospital with Becky for three months. It was heartbreaking, but it made me happy to be able to be there and hold her hand. In the beginning, the doctors would always tell us what we didn't want to hear. There were so many stages she had to get through. She had a lot of medications pumping to keep the vessels open. Because I was there every day, I was able to keep up with all that was being done for her. I knew all the medications she was taking. If they changed a dose or a medication, I would ask why. I was the type they hated. They knew I wanted to know everything that was going on and why. I'm not sorry for demanding to know everything. I wasn't able to return to work until I knew she was safe at home with family and friends who would look after her. I knew they would let me know immediately if I was needed.

How did it feel helping Becky with her therapies?
It felt as if I was helping her start over. Like a child, she had to learn from the beginning how to walk, talk, dress, eat, and so on. There were times when she wanted to give up, but I wouldn't let her. I wanted her to know I was trying to help. It was hard for me because I knew how independent she had always

been. Although she might get angry, I believed it was best for her to keep trying.

How did her personality change after her aneurysm?
The doctor warned me she might be different after recovery. He said she could be ill tempered or physically violent; however, she is even sweeter now than she was before. She was usually good natured and empathetic, but now she is extremely friendly. She shows no restraint when she is happy, excited, or pleased about something—for example, babies, animals, food, friends, and music. She is much more uninhibited in public.

She loves to sing; she is nearly always joyful. She is rarely sad or angry. She never cries but is very empathetic.

How long has it been since she has had a seizure?
She has not had a seizure since July 2015. She continues to take antiseizure meditation.

What helped you get through all those challenges?
I have a large support group: my family, my friends, and especially my sister. I am not religious, but a friend of mine is very spiritual and made me a couple of altars. I used them a lot in the beginning and continue to use them when I need to. When she was in the hospital, some friends and family members went to a crystal store, where we bought several crystals. We placed them, along with a written explanation of the significance of each crystal, into a cute bag, which I keep with me always. I am very lucky to have such supportive friends and family. They were always there for me. I was surprised that even casual friends reached out. It has meant a great deal to me.

How did your relationship with Becky change?
We were equal partners in every way before. Now, I need to take care of her. I worry about her all the time. I want to know she is safe and cared for when I can't be with her. Although she gets upset with my constant concern, I worry that some unforeseen thing could happen. Little by little she is becoming

more independent. She spends a lot more time alone now. She showers, cleans, cooks, and walks the dog without my assistance or presence. I used to be able to travel alone to visit family and friends, but now I have to make special arrangements to leave her home alone. Friends and neighbors have keys to check on her. She has to rely on others to take her places, which makes her feel so dependent.

I believe we still love and care for each other as before, but there is more worry and responsibility for me. Little by little, as she does more and more, I can relax and feel better about her regained independence.

We watched out for each other, but I was more careful about some things. For example, she wouldn't lock the door, and I would tell her, "You don't live in Iowa anymore."

Have your goals changed?
Yes. We had planned to get an RV and travel throughout the United States. Now she doesn't want to do that. Because our finances have changed, we can no longer spend freely or maintain some assets we have. We are considering selling some things, such as the motorcycles. We have to be more careful with money, and we may not be able to do some of the things we expected to do.

What is different about Becky now?
She is not able to do some things she did for me before, but she is doing more and more all the time. She does laundry, changes the sheets, does light housekeeping, waters outside, walks Jack, our dog, locks up the puppies, and cooks some meals. She is always concerned about my wellness and worries I am working too hard. She wants us to save money, so she uses coupons from the Sunday paper. She goes a little overboard. She is very proud about saving money and doesn't realize that it doesn't save us anything if we don't need or use something. I don't want to discourage her, because it is her way of taking care of me. She wants to do the shopping to save me time and effort. She feels the more independent she is, the more she is caring for me.

What has been the biggest challenge taking care of Becky?
The biggest challenge has been going back to work. That is still really hard for me. I haven't been able to go to work without thinking about her. I've had to arrange for people to be there when I was not able to. I've had to leave her in the care of others and haven't been able to be in control of everything. It has been extremely difficult to rely on others and allow them to take care of her when I would rather be there with her. I have had to trust others to protect and care for her. I haven't thought anyone else could do as well as I could with her care. I have felt I was the only one that could take care of her, but I know that is not true, which has been a great challenge to accept.

It takes more time and planning to do everything. She gets tired very easily, so we have to consider that when we go somewhere. We may not be able to stay as long or go as far away as we used to. She may need to nap during visits away. We used to sing together a lot; now she listens more. We used to take trips by car and share driving; now we have to fly, so we can't visit family as often. She doesn't like noise or loud music anymore, so we avoid some of the concerts we used to enjoy. We go to quieter, more intimate events now. We used to drink more when we went out, but now she doesn't drink. We used to talk more about everything. Now, it takes longer for her to express herself, and sometimes she stops talking because she is frustrated or tired. I have to be more patient and give her more time to express herself. Sometimes I have to help her say some things without putting words in her mouth.

Does Becky notice that?
She is very aware that we have to do things differently. She certainly notices the changes we have had to make, but she doesn't seem to mind napping in front of others when she needs to or staying home more. She consciously moves more carefully and always lets me know when she has had enough stimulation or exercise and needs to rest. Although it is difficult for her to speak, she understands most everything and is aware of everything. She doesn't want to be talked to or treated like a baby, so the differences in what we do are related to her stamina and speech difficulties. She is friendlier than ever. She is very fearless and more about taking care of business. Although it is difficult,

she deals with doctors without the help of anyone. She is appropriate in her behavior although a little more enthusiastic than before.

Do you have any advice for family members of stroke survivors?
Take one day at a time. For me it was literally minute by minute and hour by hour for a long time. Document as much as you can; take pictures and videos, and keep a scrapbook. She loves looking back and seeing improvements. Push them even though they don't want to be pushed. Tell them to do one more, read one more sentence, and have fun. One of the therapists told me to be a wife instead of a caretaker. Try to trust others to help, because it is too much for one person to do. Don't treat them like children. Try to do as many of the things you used to do as possible. Be very patient, and give them time to express themselves. Let them do as much as they can even though it takes longer and isn't perfect.

Commentary

Both Kathleen (chapter 4) and Becky's mother, Mama Bear, felt that their family members had better care because they, as advocates, demanded it. Many other families have had the same insight: all patients after a stroke need an advocate.

Part III

WERNICKE'S APHASIA

*Pearls are what oysters do about irritation. We do find
ingenious ways to compensate for life's irritations.*

—GEORGE VAILLANT, *TRIUMPHS OF EXPERIENCE*

Wernicke's aphasia is considered a receptive aphasia—that is, understanding language is a greater problem than motor speech. Individuals with Wernicke's aphasia are fluent; they use six to nine words per sentence. They can be hyperfluent, speaking very fast, often using words that are not what they intended. These word errors are paraphasias, which can be related in sound or meaning to the word they intended. The most severe errors may be nonwords, called neologisms.[28] Some individuals with Wernicke's can read orally but have difficulty writing.

The following two stories are from J and Chuck, group members who have Wernicke's aphasia.

---

28 A neologism is a new word that is coined especially by a person affected with aphasia, is meaningless except to the coiner, and is typically a combination of two existing words or a shortening or distortion of an existing word.

Eleven

J: Closer to God

J was an executive at Wells Fargo Bank before his stroke. He comes from the Philippines, and his primary language is Tagalog; he speaks a dialect of Ilocano. He left the priesthood to marry Grace. He has one daughter and a large extended family. He recently passed his driver's license test and drives one hour each way to attend our weekly Sentence Structure Group.

J is a genteel man. He is an elegant dresser and is refined in his manner and speech. He had his stroke at age sixty-one and constantly asks questions about what happened to him. He is most bothered by his inability to understand what is said and often thinks something is wrong with his hearing. He has great difficulty understanding auditory speech but does much better with written language and reads quite well. His aphasia has affected both his speech and understanding of English and Tagalog.

This is his story.

How did your stroke occur?
I was under a lot of stress both because of my work and because of my life. My mother died at the beginning of August 2014, and two nights later my brother died. On August 4, 2014, I started to slur my words, and I had a headache.

So I said to my wife, "There's something wrong with me." So we went to the Kaiser Hospital in Vallejo.

The doctor said that I should stay there for five days. I was having a stroke, and it was complicated by my diabetes. I saw a neurologist, who said there's something wrong with the left side of my brain. That part of my brain was dead.

After five days I went home, but I still had a pain in my head. So I went back to Kaiser, and they said nothing had changed, but they gave me some more medicine. I was treated for three months at Kaiser for speech therapy, and then I was cut off.

Did you get therapy after you left the hospital?
A lady at Kaiser told me about the speech group at UCDMC. So I joined the group headed by Dr. Christine Davis. I've learned a lot from that group. I thought I was having a hearing problem, but Dr. Davis told me that I could hear OK. Instead, I had a problem with auditory comprehension, which was a consequence of aphasia.

Was your family involved?
My wife and my daughter were there to support me. My wife has been a very good help. But sometimes when we talk, she'll get mad at me because she can't understand me. I want to talk more clearly so that she can understand me. But my wife and I have been closer since the stroke. My wife has had a lot of stress from her work. We don't have much money, but we are thankful for what we have. And we have faith in God. Sometimes my wife and I just pray together, and that makes us happy.

How has the stroke changed you?
I have great difficulty with communication. When I try to talk, I can hear my voice inside my head, but it doesn't come out of my mouth. When I try to talk, when I try to write, when I try to read, there's something going on in my head, but I can't write it or speak it or read it. Even when I write a name, I

write the wrong name. When somebody talks to me, I can't understand what he or she is saying. It's very frustrating.

I'm closer to God because of my stroke. Sometimes, when I was so busy at work and with everything else in my life, I forgot about God. But I am thankful and grateful because a lot of people have bigger problems, and I'm thankful that I don't have those problems. It helps to be in a group. Everybody is in the same boat, and people around me know what I'm talking about.

Before my stroke I was very talkative, but now I listen more than I talk. I don't have as much confidence as before in trying to talk. Sometimes when I'm tired, I can hardly talk at all. In the Philippines, there are so many dialects, and during therapy I heard voices in my head like dialects. It's weird.

Is there anything you miss? What activities do you enjoy?
I used to be able to listen to music and carry on a conversation at the same time. I used to dance a lot. My friends used to ask me to sing. I used to be a happy guy. Before I had a stroke, I had good conversations with people, but now I just close my eyes and listen.

What are your goals now?
In addition to being able to talk, I want to exercise more. The more you exercise, the better your brain is.

Even now, I can't believe I had a stroke. I didn't have any problems associated with a stroke. The primary problem is with my talking. There are a lot of people who are worse off because of their strokes. I think, "Hey, J, you should be grateful." I should be grateful to God that it wasn't any worse. Since I go to the Wednesday group, I see a lot of people who have it worse. Thank God I can still drive, I can still walk, and it's great.

What advice would you give to family members, caregivers, and therapists?
Be patient. Everybody should be patient. Find a stroke group like we have on Wednesdays. A group like this consists of is the only people who can understand what you've been through. Speech pathology is different from other

professions. It takes your head, your heart, and everything else. This therapy is not like a doctor, who is only interested in your body. Speech pathology is interested in your body, your mind, and your heart. Speech pathologists care about their patients and also need to be good to themselves so they can be a good person for their patients.

Commentary

J has receptive aphasia; his ability to express himself verbally is far better than his ability to understand spoken speech. Auditory language is most difficult for him to understand. He has problems processing requests with more than one step at a time; however, J reads well. J participated in an experimental verb-training program at UCDMC. This was an ideal program for him because it was computer based and did not require any auditory listening. He had to read a phrase and pick out the answer or target from a field of four pictures. Over the course of treatment, J became more efficient at learning the new verbs that were given to him. J prided himself in performing well. J now says about himself, "[My career] made me narrow, and added to that my time at Wells Fargo, I became narrow [and] not as well rounded."

Today

It was a big triumph for J to gain his driving license. He now drives the one hour to group and has no mobility problems. He plays golf and recently was happy to meet someone on the golf course who, like him, also has language problems after a stroke. Speech is still a challenge for him, especially understanding what is said to him.

Amazing Grace: J's Wife

Members of the group call her Amazing Grace because she brings us delicious treats for our Wednesday group meetings. But J's wife is amazing in other ways. J could not work at Wells Fargo after his stroke. Two months later, J's wife was laid off from her job. Instead of getting a caretaker to take care of J, his wife decided to take care of him herself. That meant she and J had to live on a very limited income. J's wife learned to manage their budget and find resources such as community food banks to supplement their limited income. J's wife says she and J rely on prayer to make their lives meaningful. Their belief in God not only holds them together in a time of crisis but also improves their spirits.

Would you describe the circumstances surrounding J's stroke?
We went to the hospital when J started having headaches and slurring his words. He was very confused. He couldn't say his name or date of birth, and then, after two days in the hospital, he had a stroke. He started saying, "You're not my wife!"

He came home five days after admission to the hospital, but he continued to complain of headaches. He called the hospital advice nurse, who asked, "What is your level of pain from one to ten?" J said ten, the max. He was in a lot of pain. He said to me, "Lay your hand on my head." He felt hot to touch. When I laid my hand on top of his head, the pain went away.

How were his spirits when he came home from the hospital?
J had great difficulty with his speech. He kept saying I was stupid. I understood, but what could I do?

How is he in public?
He doesn't say much. He's embarrassed because he can't say words right or talk perfectly. He has no signs of a stroke now, so people think he's OK. He doesn't have any physical impairments or anything like that, so we walk a lot. Our walks can take us to the outlet mall. But he doesn't want to mingle with the people we meet there. I tell him he has to practice his speech and he has to

mingle with other people. J is fretful and just says he cannot express himself well enough yet.

How does your daughter react to J?
J had his stroke when our daughter was eighteen. She gets mad at him and says she can't understand my husband. Even though J always tells his daughter, "I love you," she says, "Daddy doesn't like me." He was always very strict with his daughter. Now she wants to live at home, but she also wants to have her freedom. It's hard to negotiate both sides with J and our daughter.

Has his personality changed since he had a stroke?
No. He has always been strict with his daughter, and he is good to me. His belief in God comforts and sustains him.

Today
Grace accompanies J on the drive to group. She is constantly using community resources to make ends meet. She is an enormously generous person.

Twelve

THE FLY-FISHERMAN: FLY-FISHING THROUGH RECOVERY

Chuck is a tall, elegant, well-dressed man. He was raised in the mountains of Georgetown, learned to fish at age five, and has been fly-fishing for seventy-five years. He had a stroke while on a fly-fishing trip in the Trinity Alps at age eighty-two. His fishing partner noticed Chuck was, strangely, wobbling in the stream and losing his balance. They drove home, with Chuck driving the three hours from the Northern California stream until his fishing partner forced him to pull over so he could take over. Chuck doesn't remember driving. Once he arrived home, his wife took him to the hospital immediately.

Chuck exudes a self-confidence some find off-putting. But Chuck simply doesn't care what other people think. He has Wernicke's aphasia, which means he has great difficulty understanding written or oral directions. His speech is riddled with buzzwords and neologisms. These are actually nonwords that have some of the sounds of the target word, such as *encovertry* for *discovery*. When encouraged to slow down, Chuck can read almost flawlessly. He drives himself very hard every day. He does language activities on the web for at least two hours a day and also does physical exercises. Did I mention that he is in his eighties?

Here is his story.

What was your profession?
I was in the California Department of Boating administration.

Did you have any family history of stroke?
No, none. My mother and father were in their nineties when they died.

Did you have any symptoms before your stroke?
Yes, I did. The doctor didn't know that I was very steady on my feet. I went casting on the American River. As I was casting, I fell down. I folded in my arms, and I fell on my whole face. I thought I saw a white flock of birds and a zip zip, like a big Z. After I told my doctor, I realized that I was seeing things and hearing things that weren't there. I think the doctor was not good, because he didn't link my symptoms to a stroke.

Were you a little scared?
Yeah, I was so scared that I called the doctor, but he did not do anything about it. This happened to me a couple times previous to my stroke. I told him one time about the ziggy ziggy things. When I fell on the river, I called him up, and he gave me medicine. I carry that medicine with me, and when I get dizzy, I use it. I went to the doctor three times, telling him that I had a problem before the stroke. The doctor did not know that this was a symptom of an impending stroke. I have never had problems with cholesterol. It has always been perfect.

The doctor sent me to take a cholesterol test twice. His concern about this actually scared me. They did the test for a blockage in my carotid arteries. They have an MRI machine that goes around and makes a loud banging sound. The first MRI was a couple of weeks before the stroke and then again a couple weeks after the stroke. They both showed good results. He had me do an MRI before that summer. The gal said we can't do it again until three years have passed. After the stroke, the guy said he saw my arteries and that they were so bad that they needed to put in stents to open them for an adequate blood flow. They cut the arteries so there is good flow. I asked the guy why the first MRI came out good but my carotids are so bad. He said the plaque can be anywhere in your body.

Did you have your carotid arteries cleaned out?
No, nobody felt they had a reason to clean them before, because they felt they were all clean. Right after my stroke, I had an operation to clean them out, and then the guy said they are all bad when I had the stroke. Before my stroke everybody said all was good. They looked at the MRI, and it was perfect. Then after my stroke, he said it was terrible.

How did you know you were having a stroke?
I had a stroke while up fishing on the Trinity River. I lost my balance, and then while walking along the bank, my friend Chris said, "You don't look good. Let's rest." Then he said we have to leave. I lost my balance but did not fall down. I just felt dizzy. He told me, "You better sit down for a little bit." He felt it was more serious, so he said, "Let's go home." I actually drove back for a while, and then I told my friend that he'd better drive.

What were your symptoms during the stroke?
I was dizzy, and then it got worse and worse. Once we got home from fishing, my wife was there. She said, "Let's get out of here right now!" Then she called the fire department. I do a lot of fishing, and all of the firemen know my wife and me, so when she called, they were there in ten minutes. My wife was following. I don't remember anything after getting to the hospital. I did not see anything that I can remember.

What was happening inside your head when your friend Chris told you something was wrong with you?
Well, I knew something was going on. I never get scared. I did not realize it was a stroke at the beginning—I had no idea. Both doctors said that if your wife hadn't got you to the hospital fast, I would not have made it. When I first got home from fishing, I felt I looked pretty good, but my wife said, "You

need to get to the hospital now." When I got to the hospital, things got worse. I am not sure when I woke up, but my wife was there the whole time. All the doctors said the best thing to do is get to the hospital right away.

When did you start remembering?
I don't remember if I was in the intensive care. Probably took me a couple of days to start remembering.

What did you do to recover?
I didn't talk at all at first. I couldn't work on my speech at the hospital. I am not kidding. I would give the girls See's candies so they would let me out of the hospital. I did not really talk, just a little bit here and there, and I was not able to read.

I am a type-A person. I work out every day; I was up and working at eleven a.m. and then work out at the gym for two hours. Then I get into my [computer] programs. I have lots of them, and they are very expensive. I keep to that schedule every day. I work quite a lot.

So, when you had the stroke, nothing was wrong with your body?
My legs were weak, so I exercise them. Right now, the problem is just my talking. I tell myself whether I am good or not, and right now I am not.

Were you receiving any therapies?
I got funding for speech therapy. They paid for it after my stay in the hospital. SW's daughter was my speech therapist for a while,[29] but she had to move to Portland. I also had to leave because the money only lasted for six months. I had speech therapy an hour a day, and I got better.

What was the best part of therapy?
I am pretty good at mathematics and calculus. I liked working with math and equations.

---

29 See chapter 13.

Do you remember some of your goals?
Not too much reading at the hospital. At Mercy, they did more motor exercises. I used to work on vocabulary, but not anymore. I did not have to go to physical therapy. I went to my doctor, and he said go to speech therapy and the physical therapy. He said I need physical therapy. I would go with a therapist into a room with a bunch of like six other patients. The therapist tells me that he has a bunch of things for me to do. He wanted to evaluate where I should be in my therapy. Then he said he couldn't do anything more for me.

My doctor caught me and asked me if I was having physical therapy. I said no, and he called and asked them, "Why aren't you seeing my patient?" Then I went over there, and they told me, "I know your doctor wants me to [work with you], but there is nothing I can do for you." I told my doctor, "I don't think I need that anymore." Then the doctor told me to forget about it.

What has been your biggest challenge?
Well, the biggest challenge for me and for all that I do is to do it perfectly fine, whether it is exercising my legs or anything else. My heart and everything physical is in very good shape. The big thing I have trouble with is talking right here. The arteries were blocked, and it was my own fault; I ate and drank everything. I thought I did not have any cholesterol problems. But my arteries were clogged. It was just the arteries.

What did you learn about yourself after your stroke?
I sure learned a lot about myself, and well, I'm pretty good. I am comfortable, and I get done what I need to get done. I do not do things with other people. My wife and I do a lot of things together now. I learned that I want to know more about people. Like going to dinner and drinking a cocktail with a guy that does not know me. When he starts to talk to me, I used to say, "Who is this guy?" but now I want to talk to him. I am more appreciative.

Do you feel closer to your spouse and family?
I have two grandkids and one daughter. My wife is very helpful, and sometimes I do try to talk to her. I'm glad we understand each other. I would say,

"Look, I am sorry," and she would tell me that even if I smell or anything or curse, she knows it is part of dealing with the effects of a stroke. We have been together for forty years.

Who was with you in your recovery?
My wife and daughter. My daughter is with the State Department, and she travels with her husband. They come here every two years. They are in Africa right now.

What did they do after your stroke?
My daughter was not here. They were in Africa. I told them to not come, because it was already done.

Have you learned anything about your family or friends?
Yeah, they were so kind, and I have good friends.

Have you improved over the years following your stroke?
Yeah, from walking and reading. I exercise every day. I hop over boulders in the river.

What are your future goals?
My goal is to improve my speech, reading, and spelling.

What would be your advice for anyone who has had a stroke?
I would say two things. First, get to the hospital as fast as you can. Number two is work, work, and work to improve yourself. Look for things to fix. For me, I know what I've got to do. One thing that you need to do is to think how to do something and then do it. I did not have any physical limitations after the stroke. I do make myself talk and to do things that need to be done. I just do it. I am pretty strong. I wouldn't tell you to do anything. I am not a doctor, but I would say to keep doing what you used to do before the stroke. I do everything that I used to do before the stroke. I work on my spelling. I work really hard.

What would you tell family members?
You need to be patient with yourself, and the family members need to be patient.

What advice would you give to therapists or students?
You must have good lessons plans and have people do it. Lots of times when people talk in group, they say, "Oh, it is your turn." So, the same person answers the questions. Sometimes people are not fast. I think talking and reading are the ways to improve.

Any other feelings on your situation?
A lot of people ask me how I felt. My relationship with my family did not change. I tell people that I am friendlier. I do care a lot for people. Most of my friends are very close; they are good people. My wife and I—we do things that we like to do; we don't really do things with people if I don't know them. I came into the group wondering what I should get out of the Sentence Structure Group that will help me. You have to consider yourself. I mostly do things by myself. I used to go fishing with friends, but now I just fish by myself. I still keep in touch with my best friend, Chris.

The doctor said that because my wife got me to the hospital fast, [I did well]. Every doctor tells me that the faster you get there, the better. Have someone take you. I think it was great for me to get there right away.

Commentary

Chuck's language is a good example of Wernicke's aphasia. Chuck keeps working on his language skills about two to four hours a day. He uses a website called Talk Path. He also uses BrainHQ and Lumosity (see Appendix A, Resources). His utterances are usually very lengthy, and many words are neologisms, or nonwords, that contain parts of the word he intended to say. Chuck can sometimes catch his nonwords, and he is very persistent, repeating the word with alterations until he nails it!

Today

Chuck does mostly what he did before his stroke. That has been his goal. He goes to the gym to work out and down to the river to fly-fish. He travels to fly-fish with his friend. Although he has traveled to Africa to visit his daughter and her family since his stroke, he says those days are behind him. He enjoys brain games or anything that expands his mind. He never quits. However, sometimes he arrives to group exhausted because of the brain games he's played that day. To relax, he goes out to dinner several times a week with his wife.

Rosemary, Her Husband's Best Friend

Tell me what happened when Chuck had a stroke, from your perspective.
We were standing in our driveway talking, and all of a sudden, he started talking gibberish, and I thought, "Uh-oh!" I told him, "You better sit down." He was kind of swaying when he was talking. So, then I called 911, and the firefighters came and took him to the emergency room. He went into surgery and then went to rehab, and I don't remember how long he was there. He was in Mercy General, which is very close to where we live. He had been up out of the Trinity Alps fishing, quite a long way away. He was very lucky he had his stroke when he got back. He was up fishing with Chris, his best friend.

I followed the ambulance in the car. I was in the ER by myself. I'll never forget that a janitor took my hand and patted me. He said, "It is going to be all right."

How has life changed for you?
It hasn't changed a whole lot. He does his own thing since he is so mobile. He has not left town to fish since. He and I went to Africa to see our daughter, but he said he would never do that again. Other than his speech, I can understand him. Life goes on. I go to work, and he goes to the gym. He is more active than I am. We are not real social. Just the two of us.

At the time of the stroke, I called my daughter. She wanted to come home, but she was so far away in Africa. They do come home every summer. She has our oldest granddaughter. It was so funny to see Chuck exercising in the backyard with our eight-year-old granddaughter.

What advice would you give to spouses in your position?
Be very understanding, be calm, and don't react to how strange things are now. I actually experienced this before. My brother had a stroke and was paralyzed on the left side. He lashed out, and he was mean. I was thankful that Chuck isn't mean. I told him he is actually nicer now. You have to be calm, go with the flow. Don't let the little things bother you. We laugh a lot.

How about Chuck's friendships?

He has maintained his friendship with Chris. Chris has a full-time job raising his granddaughter, but they talk. They are fishing buddies. Chuck has been fly-fishing for over seventy-five years, since he was five years old.

Part IV

MIXED APHASIA

Hope is a thing with feathers.

—EMILY DICKINSON

Mixed aphasias are those aphasias that defy typical classification. These stories are from three individuals who have aphasia, but whose etiologies[30] are from either a tumor or anoxia rather than stroke. Two of these individuals have difficulty finding words efficiently when they talk. As a result, there are often long delays during their speech while they are searching for a word. Neither produce phonemic paraphasic errors—that is, they do not typically use words that have errors in sound or pronunciation, such as *encovery* for *discovery*. Both do, however, produce literal paraphasic errors—that is, they use words that are in the same category of the word they intended to say. For example, they might say *watch* when they mean *bracelet*. Both can have moments of fluent speech but usually require cues or assistance to complete their thoughts. Both read well and can write legibly. The third has fewer word-finding problems but does have dysarthria—difficulty producing clear speech due to ataxia—which affects his production of sentences and the intelligibility of his speech.

Three group members have mixed aphasia: Steve, Danny, and Sarbjeet. Here are their stories.

---

30 An etiology is the cause of a condition.

Thirteen

THE ENIGMA: FEW WORDS, MUCH MEANING

Steve dons a cap, usually of a fly-fishing or birding nature. He's an avid outdoorsman. He also loves to read and watch alternative films. He is mostly bald and until recently could have stood in for Santa. Unlike most of the others', his aphasia is from a brain tumor "the size of a grapefruit," as his sister says. Once the tumor was excised, a portion of his left temporal lobe was removed, resulting in aphasia. When asked a question, he more often than not replies, "I could say it yesterday or tomorrow. I know it, but I just can't say it now."

Steve was an English teacher and a newspaper reporter. He was fluent in four languages, including Russian and Mandarin Chinese. He has four children. He had sudden onset of language problems at age sixty-seven while he was teaching in an adult school in Visalia, California.

This is Steve's story.

When did you realize you had a tumor?
Before my brain tumor was diagnosed, I felt things gradually slowing down. I was teaching at an adult school in Visalia, California. On May 4, 2007, the assistant principal at school saw that something was wrong with me and took me to the hospital. I was in surgery for eleven hours; after that I was in intensive care for three days. All told, I was in the hospital for about a week and a half. I was treated very well by the nurses and hospital staff.

Was your family involved?

I have four children, two girls and two boys. They came to visit me right away. My oldest son, Casey, lives in Sacramento. He insisted that I go to Sutter Hospital, in Sacramento. So I got to ride in a small airplane to Sacramento from Visalia.

I was transferred from Sutter Hospital to Mercy Hospital. I spent six weeks at Mercy Hospital in Sacramento. I remember having speech therapy at Mercy and other kinds of therapy. Ironically, Sarah, my daughter, was a candidate for the speech-therapy master's degree program at the time. She helped me regain my speech.

I never moved back to Visalia. I moved to Sacramento to be near my son and my daughter, the one who's a speech therapist.

Has the tumor changed you in any way?

The tumor has changed my personality. Before, I was outgoing, and now I am much more introverted. I am absolutely closer to my family. My daughters, sons, and sisters and brothers—we all became closer after my tumor.

How about the Sentence Structure Group?

In the group, everybody is in the same boat. We all have aphasia. But we all are different. I had a brain tumor, so I am unlike most people, who had a stroke. Some of us are young, and some of us are old.

What activities do you enjoy? Is there anything you miss?

I like to bird-watch and take pictures of scenery. So I am excited to continue bird-watching and taking pictures. I just want to improve and live my life. I want to remember names better. I used to be good at remembering names, but after I had a brain tumor, it is not so good.

Commentary

Steve's speech characteristics are most like Broca's aphasia. He often cannot find the words he wants to say, and the length of his sentences is less than six words. He has great difficulty understanding directions that are lengthy or complex. He reads voraciously.

He is an enigma, a puzzle. Formerly a multilinguist, he spoke Russian, Mandarin, Spanish, and English before his tumor resection. He has difficulty with words but surprisingly comes up with Spanish translations of concepts we are discussing in group. He demonstrated once to the group that he could still write Mandarin characters (see below). In Mandarin, each ideographic character represents a single concept and is usually spoken as a pitched monosyllable, or single syllable. For example, the monosyllable *ma*, depending on its pitch upward or downward, can change meaning from "horse" to "mother" or frame the sentence as a question.

A man of few words, Steve nevertheless imbues his sentences with meaning. Recently he came to the group with a book tucked under his arm titled *Kafka*. When I asked what word described this book, Steve said, "Despair."

Today

Steve takes pictures, mostly of nature, birds, and scenery. He loves films and reading. Steve is ingenious; he makes his own laundry soap. He's living the good life every retired person wants—except he can't drive, but this doesn't concern him. He travels by train or air instead and locally walks or takes public transportation.

Steve's Writing of a Sentence in Spanish and "I Am" in Mandarin Characters

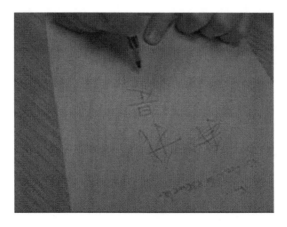

Alice, also known as Steve's Pesky Little Sister

When did you realize Steve had a tumor?
Steve had gained a lot of weight and was depressed. I was very concerned about him. The tumor was growing, and none of us knew anything about it. He was teaching English as a second language when he had his first symptoms of the brain tumor. Steve told his students another teacher was going to come and teach so he could go home. The teacher then went over to Steve's house to see how he was doing. You know how Steve jokes around. They thought he was just joking but then realized he was really sick. They took him to the hospital that night. We didn't have any clues this was going on. His tumor was the size of a grapefruit, and it took an eleven-hour surgery to remove it. That is why he has a scar on the side of his forehead. For six months he had to wear a blue helmet, which also had some pads to protect his skull. He went through a lot.

Tell us a little bit about his upbringing.
Steve and I both were raised in a military family. There were three generations of military people in our household in New Mexico. Both our grandfathers, paternal and maternal, were colonels. Our maternal grandfather lived with us in Las Vegas, New Mexico. Our father was a retired major and graduate of West Point.

Steve is very bright and was reading books at the age of five. When he was in third grade, he was reading *A Tale of Two Cities*. He is a huge reader. But he was bored in school. He acted out a lot because the teachers could not give him enough to do. Perhaps because we grew up in a military family, Steve never liked authority.

At eighteen, Steve volunteered to serve in the Vietnam War. The military sent him to the naval language school to learn Mandarin. He was self-taught in Spanish and learned Russian. He was always good at languages.

What happened after he had a brain tumor?
Eventually he recovered pretty well. He lost his facility with languages, but he remembers phrases, especially in Spanish.

How has that affected your relationship?
He is my big brother and would always tease me. Now we do a lot together, so we are pretty close.

How well can he communicate with you?
I try to challenge him. I speak slowly, but I don't give him words. He'll say, "I have the words in my head, but I can't tell you things that I want to say to you." We recently went to the Apple store, and they spoke so fast that he was confused. That's so sad because he was great with words and language. But he never complains and just loves everybody.

What does he do now?
He doesn't drive anymore, but he lives downtown, so many activities are convenient for him. He reads a lot of books and goes to many movies. He enjoys photography and bird-watching. He's perfect with his identification of birds.

Fourteen

HAPPY-GO-LUCKY: WHEN AM I GOING TO GET MY DAMN LICENSE?

*D*anny has the mannerisms of a southern gentleman. His speech is slow, and he often takes his time, looking up, trying to figure out how to put his thoughts into words. He is a devoted husband to his wife, Peg, who looks after him. If he is home late, she calls the hospital to make sure he hasn't gotten lost or missed Paratransit. They are a great couple. Danny had a grand mal seizure in 2011 before they discovered his tumor. Four years later he had a stroke.

Here is his story.

Tell us about your stroke.
I had one grand mal seizure back in Ohio when I went to my daughter's graduation. I went home, took a nap, and had a seizure. They transferred me from the top of her apartment building down to the bottom floor, and there were eleven kinds of twists and turns. Transporting me from the top floor was not so good. The next thing I knew, I was in the hospital. When I saw my doctor, he just said that I was in pretty bad shape. I was probably in the hospital five days. I got home, and I rested for a while with bandages on my head. My speech was not impaired. I didn't feel like I was going to die; I just felt sore all over and dizzy.

I then had a stroke, which was pretty bad. I remember I called my wife from home and I mentioned to her that my right arm and my left hand were failing. She got home from work, and we went to the urgent care. Well, first we went to the doctor's office; then we went to the emergency care. That is when all the things happened—the speech and everything else.

What were the symptoms of your stroke?
There was still a lot of pressure in my brain. Once the doctors took care of that, then I had to go to Sutter Memorial to see more experts. I had bandages on my head because they had to operate in order to relieve the pressure on my brain.

How was your experience at the hospital?
When I was released from Sutter General, they transferred me to Roseville for rehab. Well, they kept waking me up. All they did was wake me up. My family was able to visit me, and all of my grandkids came to visit me.

Did you have any therapies?
Yeah, I had treatments for my brain. I had speech therapy, MRIs, and had physical therapy.

How did you feel after your stroke?
I didn't get depressed before the stroke. But I did quit working and so retired. My wife has always been there to support me, and my two daughters have always been there too. There are eight and a half years in between each daughter. My relationship with my daughters changed. One of my daughters lives close to me, and she has four kids. They have always been close to us for the most part. I have a younger brother, who lives in Oregon, and he comes down just to visit me. My wife is my main support.

Tell us about your therapy.
It was OK, and it couldn't have been better. Everything that my therapist did for me was OK. I remember this speech therapist, and she tried to get me to

say something. I was able to say a little bit. I don't recall the first words I said after the stroke.

What was your biggest challenge after the stroke?
Initially, I had the OK from my doctor to get a driver's license. Now, however, one of the challenges is not being able to drive. I took the driver's test. But that is not either here or there. I am not that concerned with my speech, because it was more my independence that I wanted.

How has your stroke impacted you?
It's not really all that bad. I just have a limp on my right foot, and I can't move my right hand that much. I have always liked to read picture books, and I don't have any problems with that. I like to go for a walk for entertainment. I used to play golf, but I don't play golf anymore. My youngest daughter is still living at home, and she has a job and can be messy but is very helpful. I don't feel that the stroke has brought anything negative into my personality. I have always had the personality of saying few words, and I feel that I still have that same personality. I am taking a lot of medications. Monday, Wednesday, and Friday, I have a person at home that watches over me. Tuesday and Thursdays, I'm by myself. No caregiver since July.

What did you do before your stroke?
I wanted to do business in the food industry. I have always been a cake sales-man. I started out with the grocery business, then went to Dolly Madison, and then to Hostess. I have always been in the grocery business. I think that one of the things is that everybody's got to eat.

Do you have any goals?
I would want to talk in full sentences. I don't have any therapies, but I attend the Sentence Structure Group. I feel that I still continue to improve. I used to use the cane a couple of years ago. Now I am more independent. I am still try-ing to get that damn license. That process is somewhere in between the nurse's office and the doctor.

I will be going on a trip in July to Alaska on a cruise. I would like to start some hobbies with my wife. For example, playing catch or going to the gym. I would like to stay active with my wife. We don't do that right now, but I would like to do that. I would like to read too. My ultimate goal is to read again. I can read only a little bit. I read the lines, and then I go back and reread what I can from the lines.

What advice would you give to other stroke patients?
Be patient and don't let it get you down. First thing I did when I got back from Ohio was start chemotherapy for my tumor, and second thing I did was to have my stroke. I spent two weeks in the hospital. The stroke was challenging. They have been all one long process. I advise people to go to groups like the one Dr. Christine Davis has. If there is one piece of advice I could give it's to go to the hospital right away.

What advice do you have for students or therapists that work with patients with stroke?
I would tell them to not give up on them [stroke patients].

Does anything worry you?
I worry about what would happen if Peg [my wife] would get sick. That is one of my biggest worries.

Commentary
So often in group, Danny will be the first one to find a word that escapes everyone else. It is so delightful when this happens because Danny is a man of so few words that he rarely utters a lengthy sentence.

Today
Danny attends the Sentence Structure Group weekly. He walks independently after some time with a walker. He does not drive. This is a sore subject for

Danny; he would really like to get his damn license back (as he says). He recently took a cruise to Alaska. He was so enthusiastic when he returned that he spoke to us at great length about his excursions and the scenery. We were all taken aback by this surge of lengthy sentences! He is an optimist and is incorrigibly cheerful.

Peg, Danny's Wife: You Need a Sense of Humor!

Who took care of Danny after his stroke?
Everyone wanted to help him. I had to work forty hours a week, from eight to five, so my daughter had someone from church take care of him for fifty-six hours a week. Now he has a caretaker only for six hours, three days a week. No caretaker since July.

Are there things he does not do anymore?
He sometimes has sensory overload and gets exhausted very fast. He gets tired more easily. We used to travel. I can't drive up into the mountains. I am very scared of heights, and Dan used to be the one to drive the Tahoe. He was very good at that and liked doing it.

Sometimes I tell him to do things, and he says no. Now I ask him, "Why don't you want to do that?" He says, "Because I do not want them to think I am slow." Some people would think it was an intellectual problem. I understand why they would think so.

Also, I have learned that when we want to go somewhere, we need to know where we are going before we get in the car. One time we got lost, so I parked the car and turned off the radio. We took deep breaths and then talked about where we wanted to go eat. Our daughter would ask, "Did you get mad at Daddy?" I would say, "I get irritated, and then I get irritated that I got irritated."

What was his biggest challenge?
He had a lot of troubles with his urinary tract and had to go through multiple procedures involving a catheter. That is a big challenge because you have to take good care of the catheter and make sure a urinary tract infection doesn't happen. Having a catheter also impacts the urinary tract, so he had to go through multiple procedures after they took the catheter away. They are going to put a pacemaker in his bladder late in October.

Did you learn anything from the stroke?
You know, we have gone through a lot of things, and I went through a lot of things prior to the surgery. I consider myself a strong woman, but I look back

to what we went through now, and I can't believe I did not lose my sense of humor. We learned to talk about how we feel. Sometimes I will tell him what makes me upset, and we will talk about it, and sometimes he will tell me what makes him upset. That has made our relationship stronger. We communicate more about how we feel now. Before, he would work, and it was a routine, the eight-to-five. Now we have the time to talk more about what we feel.

Do you have any advice for family members or professionals?
We were very blessed to have doctors that were very nice. We still have the same doctors. I am surprised that young people are very patient with him and let him take his time when ordering food. Everyone just has been very good to us.

Family members need to know a stroke is not just an event. A stroke, as bad as it is, can get worse, and sometimes it can get better. It can get worse for a minute, days, or even months. People need to understand that a stroke can get worse as time passes, that it is never at one level. When he had his stroke, Dan got worse within twenty-four hours. People think it stays at one level, but it was not that way with him.

Sometimes when his symptoms are bad, I think, "Oh no." I am scared it is another stroke.

What advice would you give to people in your situation?
To have patience. For example, people need to be more patient when they have a customer that needs more time when ordering. People in retail need to be trained in how to serve people that take a little bit more time to choose what they want or to place an order. It is very important that there be more awareness, because it is not an intellectual problem. They just have trouble getting their words out. We went to Sutter Stroke Camp, and they help spread awareness about stroke. They do the Head Trauma Support Project, and we participated in that. We learned from them, and it helped us.

Let your family member know when he or she is getting better. For example, Wednesdays are very tough days for Dan because he uses the Paratransit. One day when he got home, he told me, "The bus driver is not going to be able to come to the house. She is going to call you on the phone to reschedule." I said, "Why can't she come to the house?" and he said, "Insurance!" I told him, "You know what? Wednesdays are the toughest for you, and yet you were able to tell me everything." Even though he did have trouble naming things, he did not leave anything out.

Speech therapy is a big thing. Dan can go one week without speech therapy, and he is OK, and even two weeks without speech therapy, but after three weeks without therapy, you can really tell the difference. He gets worse. Speech therapy is very important; stroke survivors need to have consistent speech therapy.

Commentary

Peg works full time. Peg, like Kathleen (chapter 4), has found a sense of humor to be invaluable. It is a way to buoy yourself through the difficult times.

Fifteen

Conversations with God

Sarbjeet's wife just completed her second bachelor's degree. Her prior bachelor's was in education, and in 2016 she completed her degree in speech pathology and audiology and is currently applying for the master's program. She decided to pursue this program after her husband had a catastrophic heart attack that resulted in motor and speech-language deficits. Here is her story.

Thank you for agreeing to this interview.
First, I'd like you to know you are definitely making a difference in people who have had a stroke. My husband, who is not very expressive with his feelings, was recently asked to share which types of therapy have significantly helped him since his event almost five years ago. He chose his therapy group with you at UC Davis as one of the therapy experiences that has been the most meaningful. My parents have also noticed a change in his communication after his group sessions that you provide. Thank you.

Can you go over the event of your husband's heart attack?
It was February 28, 2012, around one in the afternoon, when I received the phone call. The morning had started normally. Sarbjeet had gone to work as he did each morning. I spoke to him around eleven, when he mentioned

he was going to go to the gym and was very excited to play squash with a friend who was coming from Reno. That morning, he completed his rounds in the hospital and later went to his clinic to see his scheduled patients for the morning. He played two games of squash, and according to his friend, they played particularly hard that day—something I am not surprised by. Sarbjeet often played hard, regardless of the sport. He really enjoyed being active. After playing, they both sat down for a bit next to the court. While they were sitting down, Sarbjeet's friend noticed that Sarbjeet was feeling his wrist. Those in medicine think he was feeling his pulse. His friend thought Sarbjeet was concerned about his carpal tunnel. Sarbjeet then fell over, quite suddenly. His friend thought he was playing a joke, pretending the game had been too strenuous. When the friend noticed that Sarbjeet tried to get up, lifting himself slightly, and then collapsed again, he knew it wasn't a joke and yelled for help. Two ladies, one a physician and the other a nurse from Kaiser, tried to help. They started to give him CPR. The gym manager came by and brought the AED, so they used that plus CPR. Unfortunately, it did take eight minutes for the ambulance to arrive.

The phone call I received from the manager was "Your husband has collapsed, and we are trying everything we can to revive him." I was in shock and trying not to focus on the words "trying to revive him." I got the car keys and drove to the gym. On my way to the gym, I prayed and asked God for his help!

I arrived at the gym and met the ambulance team as they were working on Sarbjeet. I recall saying, "Take him to the hospital. Take him to the hospital." The ambulance person was rude to me and simply said, "Ma'am, we are doing everything we can." Sarbjeet's friend took me aside because I just kept repeating, "Take him to the hospital."

Finally, Sarbjeet was taken to the hospital. I drove over with Sarbjeet's friend. We went to Sutter Roseville, the hospital where Sarbjeet had worked. That was good and bad. The bad was that his colleagues had to see him like this. The good was that everyone was motivated to help. The staff at Sutter Roseville was prepared; as soon as he got to the ER, they took him to the cath lab. The cardiologist was waiting for Sarbjeet at the ER. The pulmonologist told me they put him in hypothermia because he was not responding. Much later the cardiologist came and said he put a stent in and Sarbjeet had had a massive heart attack. He also told me Sarbjeet was in hypothermia and was not going to wake up for three days. That was the protocol since he was not responding. I can't remember exactly whether there was a change after the three days. He wasn't becoming more conscious. We never spoke, and I never saw any consciousness after that. They asked Sarbjeet to move his hand or wiggle his toes. Apparently, none of the physicians saw him do it. But my brother, who is also a physician, did see him respond to commands. The neurologist came during his time off and saw him responding too, but he was not able to record this in Sarbjeet's medical records, because he was just visiting that day.

Early on how were you doing? How were you feeling?
First I was in a panic. That night, when I came home, I was very hopeful. I was still shocked, but I was very hopeful. Maybe being oblivious helped me be very hopeful. I don't remember feeling he was not going to make it. I was just scared. Our youngest daughter was sixteen at the time, and she was in high school. When the cardiologist came, our daughter asked him whether her dad was going to be OK. The doctor sort of choked up and said, "I don't know, but I hope so." I told the doctor our son was in Spain as an exchange student. I asked him whether we should tell him to come back. He said yes.

At what point did he start recovering?
Sarbjeet's story is unique. One of Sarbjeet's friends, a cardiothoracic surgeon, found out about what had happened to Sarbjeet, I believe through Facebook. He called me and asked me to describe what happened and then said he would call me later. He called me later and asked me to send him Sarbjeet's EEG reports, which showed his frequent seizures. He then said to me his neurologist friend looked at Sarbjeet's EEG and said Sarbjeet was a textbook case. He said Sarbjeet needed medication to make his seizures stop. The friend spoke with Sarbjeet's neurologist and found out the medication had not yet been administered. The friend then flew out from New York to see Sarbjeet. It had been one week since the incident, and the pulmonologist and the neurologist wanted to meet with me. I met with them, and I had my sister come with me. We

sat down with the pulmonologist, and he said Sarbjeet was not responding. They asked me what I thought. I told them I didn't know. Just as the meeting was going to end, our MD friend from New York walked in and said, "So are you guys going to do the procedure?" The pulmonologist and neurologist both asked about the procedure and gave mixed responses; the pulmonologist responded that it was fine, and the neurologist asked to be removed from the case.

Luckily, we had a friend in town who was also a neurologist. The procedure Sarbjeet would be given included administering medications to control the seizures and put him in a coma. He was already sort of in a coma since he was not responding, but this was an induced coma. The next day the neurologist took the case, and shortly after, Sarbjeet was induced into another seventy-two-hour coma. After the coma, they told us they were going to watch and see how he responded. Unfortunately, there wasn't much change in Sarbjeet's status. I remember one night when I returned from the hospital, my parents and siblings were trying to discuss Sarbjeet's condition in the most sensitive way they knew and the options for moving forward the physicians had presented. That was when I started thinking maybe he wouldn't make it. However, I really didn't want to make the decision. I felt awful. I don't remember thinking even once about what to do, now two weeks into this ordeal. I felt the most pressure about having to make a decision about Sarbjeet's life. Also, one of the physicians took me aside and told me Sarbjeet didn't want to have all the tubes, just lying there in a vegetative state. I believed him. The physician also told me it was very expensive to keep him like that in a nursing home. I remember saying we had insurance. He then told me, "Well, I wouldn't give him more than a month." I had a conversation with God, asking him to wake Sarbjeet up before the month was over. I don't remember why, but I wanted him to wake up before the end of the month.

That time in the hospital was amazing, in a variety of ways. I thought I knew everything about my husband. Yet day after day I received overwhelming support from all the people that loved Sarbjeet. I told myself, "I really don't know this guy." Everyone had a story about him. He used to tell a joke a day. On many occasions, I would see family, friends, and colleagues waiting in the conference room given to us as a waiting room. When they visited him, they would tell him how much they missed him. They would say, "Wake up and tell me a joke." They would remember he had such a loud voice that they could tell when he was coming because they could hear him in the hallways. That was so positive.

Another story I like to share is about the day I was feeling the most pressure to make a decision and I got a phone call from the technician who did his EEG. I think she was at UC Davis and had years of experience. She called me and said she was doing this off the record and if they ever asked her, she would have to deny she called me. She told me that when she did the EEG, she was 100 percent sure he moved his eyes. She knew he was there. She said she was not supposed to say anything. That was the hope I received that night. God had answered my prayers.

So how much longer was he in that state?
On March 24, there was supposed to be a big party for an organization Sarbjeet was a part of, California Sikh Foundation. Instead of the party, they decided to have a prayer for him that day. Sarbjeet woke up on the twenty-third, a day before the prayer. The Sikh community was our backbone during this traumatic event our family was going through. They held a prayer for Sarbjeet at the hospital chapel each Wednesday during his hospitalization.

When he woke up, what was that like?
That is my favorite experience I have had as his wife. It is one of those movie experiences. I went in that morning, and I was very relaxed. I went to him, and I gave him a kiss. It seemed I got a tiny response. Then I said, "Oh my God," and I asked him to give me a kiss again. Sarbjeet then puckered his lips. I told the pulmonologist, "He just gave me a kiss." I asked Sarbjeet to give me a kiss again to make sure I was not just seeing things. All the intensive care unit personnel came in and were clapping. I asked Sarbjeet to kiss me again, and he did. The pulmonologist then told him, "Stop kissing her already!"

He started to open his eyes. Family and relatives from out of town had come to visit him, and he was able to recognize everyone. After he started to respond, he went to the floor. He was trached a week after being admitted. Even though he was able to breathe, he was trached because he was not responding. However, he was able to breathe by himself.

Was he being tube-fed?
He did have a G tube.[31] On April 4, he went to Sutter Rehabilitation. He was the medical physician at Sutter Medical Rehabilitation. Can you imagine that? The story the CEO likes to tell is that Sarbjeet and his friend, who is a rehab physician, were the ones that proposed having a rehabilitation unit at Sutter Roseville Medical Center. His friend was the director of the Sutter Medical Rehabilitation when Sarbjeet was there as a patient. They were all shocked because he had seen patients at the rehab center the morning of the incident. One friend of ours says God had a plan for Sarbjeet to use the facility he proposed be built. We are so fortunate to have all these friends.

How long was he in rehab?
He was there from April 4 through May 29. He had all three therapies during his stay.

When did he start talking?
I think his first words were when the neurologist asked him, "What are you going to give a patient with a cough?" Sarbjeet responded, "Amoxicillin." I think that is what it was. That is what Sarbjeet responded when the neurologist was testing his knowledge on medicine. It happened right after the ICU.

When did he start putting words together?
This doctor that spoke Hindi walked in one day. Sarbjeet started speaking to him in Hindi. His speech was hard to understand, but he was able to communicate thoughts but not full sentences. He had the trach tube removed April 2 but had a hole there and had to cover it with his finger to talk.

---

31 G-tube is a gastrostomy tube (also called a G-tube) inserted through the abdomen that delivers nutrition directly to the stomach.

You are studying speech pathology, so from a speech and language standpoint, what was he like when he was released?
Cognition was very low in terms of memory and attention. The speech pathologist told me he was not remembering anything new. But fortunately, he surprised us one day when he asked me, "How was Whole Foods?" He had overheard me talking to some friends about going to Whole Foods for lunch. He was also having some swallowing issues. After a week of rehabilitation, he was on honey-thick liquids, and then he was on a regular diet by the time he got home. His speech was unintelligible. His expressive language was extremely limited.

What were they doing for cognition?
They were working on sequencing as well as receptive and expressive language using flash cards. I remember the therapist saying he did very well in the session I observed. He likes to perform.

When he was discharged, did he have outpatient services?
He had Rehab Without Walls because he came home with a wheelchair and a walker. He never used the wheelchair at home. He was using his walker independently in the house. He had Rehab Without Walls the day after his release until the end of August. Then he did outpatient therapy at Sutter until February 2013.

I found it very disturbing initially that Sarbjeet had just moments of clarity. Fortunately, with time those moments increased significantly. His vocabulary seems to be completely intact. His sentence length is normal when he speaks in Punjabi. However, fluency is slightly impaired because of the dysarthria. He is currently going to Sacramento State's Neuro Service Alliance therapy and UC Davis aphasia groups.

What is the most important thing for him?
He always says it is his family.

Do you think he has accepted where he is now?
I wouldn't say he is fine with it, but I think he accepts who he is right now. Sometimes I ask him what he misses the most, and he always says he misses his patients.

How are you feeling now?
I started to go to therapy. I went to an Easterseals' support group. The first year was very tough for me. I couldn't speak the whole time I was there. Somebody told me, "Don't worry. It gets better after three years." So I was sort of waiting for three years. Unfortunately, it didn't happen. I was watching TV, and somebody said, "Grief is something you don't have control over. It will come to you without notice." So I acknowledged and accepted it in the moment and let it pass. I started to practice that. I wouldn't fight it. I think that helped me.

The other thing is acceptance. I would say, "Sure, I have accepted this. I have convinced myself." And then one day I noticed that accepting the new normal changes from day to day. It isn't constant; maybe one day I have accepted it, and another I have not. Today I am very grateful that my acceptance is stronger. I am proud that I know what acceptance means. I didn't even know what that meant before. People would ask me, and I would say sure. But now I actually know what that means. It was really hard to cross that path and accept. It meant I would forget the life I had. How could I forget my past life?

It also meant that to help him improve, I no longer would hope or wish or do things for him now that I have accepted. I think I have started to improve on that. I remember that on my way to the gym when I got the news, I had a conversation with God. I remember believing and saying to myself that something good would come out of this. One day I was going to say, "This is the good." The good is I'm studying speech therapy. I would have never taken this road otherwise. Throughout this experience, the common thread is the kindness I have been fortunate to experience. I am very grateful to my parents, my siblings with their families, and our friends for the love and support they have provided unconditionally to us as we navigate this journey.

Commentary

Sarbjeet is an exception in our group. Because of his heart attack, he had anoxic brain injury—that is, a lack of oxygen to the brain—and no focal lesions, as we have seen in all other members of our group. The problems he has with speech and language are primarily motoric; the articulators and breath control for speech are affected. His speech is dysarthric or weak, meaning his articulation is slurred or imprecise and with poor breath support. As a result, his speech is often hard to understand.

His fluency, or the number of words he uses in a sentence, is in the nonfluent range (fewer than six to nine words per sentence) because he does not have the breath support to articulate a full, intelligible sentence.

Today

Sarbjeet is a renowned doctor at his medical facility. Even now he has patients waiting for him to return to practice after five years. This is a testament to his skill and compassion as a physician. He has three children, a son and two daughters. All his children are interested in pursuing premed. It seems his children are following in his footsteps.

Sarbjeet doesn't drive and has persistent balance difficulties. Family members drive him to his appointments. He attends the local university speech clinic and our Sentence Structure Group. His vocabulary is essentially intact. He is quick to insert or find a word that escapes other members of the group. He is witty and fun, a treasured member of our group.

Part V

Living with Aphasia

Pray. Not for God to cure you, but to help you help yourself.

—Kirk Douglas, *My Stroke of Luck*

This section begins with a chapter for families and stroke survivors about getting through each phase of recovery: the acute phase, rehabilitation, discharge home, and life after stroke. It also offers advice on taking care of yourself. This advice is distilled from my thirty years of work with individuals and families dealing with aphasia, including these interviews.

The next and last chapter is "Final Thoughts on Better Outcomes." This is a compilation of what I have learned, which is that people have tremendous resilience, which often surprises even them, to endure hardships and find a way to respond to life's challenges and recover their purpose and meaning. I hope you will find this section useful and enlightening.

Sixteen

What You Should Know at Each Phase of Recovery

*H*ere are nuggets of wisdom gleaned from interviewing individuals with aphasia and their families.

Things Everyone Should Know

Recognize the signs of a stroke. **Act FAST:** facial droop, arm weakness, speech slurred or strange, time to call 911.

The Earliest Phase of Recovery: The Acute Phase

This phase begins at the time of admission to the emergency ward through admission to the rehabilitation unit or discharge home, whichever comes first. Here are eight pieces of advice that apply during this phase.

- Every stroke survivor needs an advocate. As an advocate, you can be demanding. This cannot be overstressed. The medical community is hard to navigate. It is impossible for those facing new problems in expressing themselves and understanding what is said. They need their families and caregivers to advocate for them.

- Be there. Be present bedside.
- The patient may say something [hurtful] unintentionally. Don't take anything said by the patient personally.
- When communicating with the patient, use short sentences and slow speech down. Use pictures to help communicate.
- Stay calm; be positive. If you are going to cry, leave the room.
- Learn more about stroke and aphasia by asking your medical professionals. Use Google if all else fails.
- Have hope.
- Begin keeping a diary of all the information you learn from your experience and from the medical professionals. You may need to go back and review it later.

The Rehabilitation Phase of Recovery

This phase begins when patients are admitted to the rehabilitation unit or discharged home. If they are discharged home, they may have rehabilitation continued with home health therapists coming into the home. This is a time of rapid change. The brain is healing, so behavior, motor, and language skills are improving. Sometimes you will see changes from day to day.

- Make sure visitors don't stay too long. Patients are using all their resources to heal. Rest and sleep are essential for their recovery.
- Look up resources on the web.
- Recruit family and friends to help.

Life after Stroke

This phase begins when the patient leaves the rehabilitation unit or is discharged from home therapy. You may still be participating in outpatient therapy, but you are home and essentially on your own. Each family member interviewed contributed to this section, and each is given credited for his or her words of wisdom.

- People with aphasia do better if caregivers and friends speak slowly.
- Caregivers need to know the difference between helping stroke survivors and infantilizing them. Be respectful; treat them as the adults they are. (Michael)
- Get patients into a support group; it is a way for them to see they are not alone. (Jeff, Jana's husband)
- Develop a sense of humor! (Peg, Danny's wife)
- Someone needs to help organize the patient's social activities. (Jana)
- Stay connected to your family and friends; they can help you. (Kathleen, Michael's wife)
- Try to do everything you did before your stroke. (Chuck)
- Don't mourn the past or fear the future; be here in this moment. (Kathleen, Michael's wife)
- Keep them going so they feel good about themselves. (Bob, Jason's father)
- Let them struggle to say what they want to say; don't jump in to help too soon. (Kai, Michael's daughter)
- It is a matter of being patient and kind. Let them take care of the tasks they can. Give them an open door to vent feelings. Love them and expect more of them as they recover. (Bob, Jason's father)
- Consider transportation and location. The suburbs can isolate a survivor from resources such as public transportation, theaters, and easy access to events. Investigate transportation services (Paratransit, private drivers, any ADA transportation provider) so the survivor can begin to be independent.

Suggestions from Members of the Group

Michael's Suggestions

People talk so fast and move on to the next topic so fast that the stroke survivor may just give up on something he or she wants to say.

Don't be too overprotective; it may give stroke survivors a sense that they aren't going to be OK, that there's a reason to worry.

Repetition in relearning is the key. Just because stroke survivors did something once doesn't mean it "stuck." They may have trouble and need help with the same task later. Be patient.

Remember that people have brains but they don't know how to express their intelligence again yet. Don't treat them as if they were stupid or had forgotten everything they knew before their stroke.

Technology can be frustrating, especially if they used it before the stroke. Be patient.

Stroke survivors have gone through hell (well, at least a life-changing experience), and depression afterward is common and understandable. Seek professional help from your doctor or a therapist.

If you are a supporter of a stroke survivor, self-care is vital. Don't be a martyr—it will hurt both you and your stroke survivor in the long run.

If you are a spouse or a significant other, don't assume the role of therapist. It may hurt your relationship permanently. Follow the therapist's advice on this—it's critical.

Keep up the physical exercise; it's important to health and well-being.

Suggestions for People with Physical Limitations Such as Hemiparesis,[32] from Don and Linda

If a person has problems walking in a room, move furniture so there is more room for walking. Remove furniture that has sharp corners or is fragile.

If arms/hands are paralyzed or weak, when providing food, put silverware and napkins on the person's functioning side.

Open bottles of water, juice, and milk for the person. Also, use easy-open bottles.

To help with reading newspapers, open the paper and separate the pages. Put them in order on the table.

---

32 Hemiparesis is a unilateral or one-sided weakness or paresis. It can affect the left or right side of the body. It can involve the arm and leg or only one limb. *Hemi* means "half."

Put a nightlight in bathrooms and hallways to guide him or her to the bathroom at night.

Trim the person's nails and toenails.

If there are stairs in the house, have handrails installed on both sides of the stairs.

Advice for Taking Care of Yourself, the Family, Caregivers, and the Stroke Survivor from Michael *Maher.*

The stroke survivor's brain keeps healing, but don't expect him or her to heal perfectly. The person might, but he or she might not.

Accept that this is where you are now. Live life in the moment.

There is a fine line between striving to get better and being at peace with where you are now.

Pray, meditate, and find inner peace.

Stay connected with your friends; you need their support.

Be a gatekeeper. Make sure visitors don't overstay their welcome; stroke survivors tire easily and need their rest.

How to Help Stroke Survivors with Aphasia, from Jana

Here are suggestions to help a stroke survivor who experiences aphasia. My family told me these are some of the important actions they took to help me. These items helped me deal with a stroke with aphasia when I lost my ability to find words, understand, listen, read, and write. People who have physical problems may or may not need this assistance. Brain damage affects different parts of the brain. Each person responds differently. Although I think these suggestions are helpful, just ask a stroke survivor what he or she needs.

Speech therapists are excellent professionals that provide treatment and assist families and friends. Help people, who are willing to get speech therapy, and encourage them to get as much speech therapy as they can and attend as long as possible.

Be supportive of the stroke survivor. Although you may need to help her or him with many activities, show respect by not commanding the person to do something. Speak kindly even if you need to be firm.

Promote a calm and soothing attitude while you are with the stroke survivor. The person may not want to talk to many people because of overstimulation. Ask the person if he or she wants to postpone having relatives, friends, or other visitors who are high-energy people come to the hospital or home. Respect and follow the person's needs.

Let people rest and sleep, especially when they are recovering from a stroke. People need an amazing amount of rest and sleep for their brains to heal. Please don't force them into activities they are too tired to do.

Talk slowly. I suggest you talk as slowly as the person talks. That will help the brain process what is said and gives the person time to understand.

If needed, when giving information or directions, break all your actions into small steps, one or two at a time.

If you are having a conversation, wait and give the person time to talk with you. Ask the person whether he or she wants you to help finish sentences or find words and when the person does want help.

Help keep the person's home quiet if needed. Ask whether it is hard or impossible to watch TV or movies or listen to music, the radio, or other sounds. Respond accordingly.

Here are suggestions to help a person talk, read, spell, write, listen, and understand what is said. Use books, games, and toys to teach the person at his or her appropriate level after a stroke. Ask the person to list things that are important to him or her and frequently need to be communicated, such as the town where the person lives, his or her family, work, hobbies, activities, favorite food, and so on. Help the person make a picture book illustrating these things, which will help the person communicate these ideas with others.

I hope this information will be helpful to you or others who may need to help stroke survivors with aphasia.

Seventeen

FINAL THOUGHTS ON BETTER OUTCOMES

Just Showing Up

Can you imagine having had a stroke and entering a room with a group of people you've never met before? This is after you know speaking is very difficult for you. You also know this meeting was designed to make you do what is most difficult: to talk, and to talk in complete sentences. This is the room all my patients enter. Why do they show up, and why did they come in the first place?

The first component of this group is that it is safe, a safe place to talk. Participants need to feel they can trust the group facilitator and the other members of the group, with no harsh judgments, no pressure, and no expectations except that they need to show up and try.

They show up because they believe somehow this will help them achieve, if not a direct improvement in language, then an improvement in self-esteem, self-acceptance, and *hope*.

The group is the setting where participants can unload the burden of feeling alone. By showing up, participants share one another's load. They widen their views. They see others like themselves, some with better speech and some with worse. Some are at peace with themselves, and others are not. It is a matter of courage, I think, to show up and return each week. It is also a matter of hope.

After a few weeks of showing up, a new dynamic takes place. Acquaintances become friends. We get to know one another, and we wonder where you are if you don't show up. We see improvements and applaud them. We notice change, good and bad. We worry about one another. For example, Steve's speech got worse in group.[33] Even his e-mails were unintelligible. We noticed the decline, and then came the news: Steve's brain tumor had grown. We had the first inkling of this in group. He underwent surgery and is now recovering well.

Putting It in Perspective

I'm reminded of a Buddhist story. A teacher instructs his apprentice to gather his pain and sorrows in a pile, like a pile of salt. That amount of salt is your total pain and sorrow. He instructs the apprentice to put that salt in a small glass of water and drink it. It is bitter and hard to swallow. Then the teacher instructs him to put that same amount of salt in a lake. The lake represents the entirety of his life, pain and pleasure, and he drinks from the lake. Now it is sweet and refreshing. The same amount of salt, the same amount of pain and sorrow, mixed in with all the aspects of one's life makes the bitter taste sweeter.[34]

It is a matter of pulling back and looking at the entirety of your life, not just the loss or the pain. The group helps us do that. The group widens our views. And sharing seems to lessen the load.

As a trained researcher, I can't help but look for correlates of good outcome. I look around the room at the group and see that good outcomes seem to have little to do with recovery of language or the results of brain scans. The following are *observations* and not the result of scientific inquiry, but they may

---

33 See chapter 12.
34 Abstracted from Mark Nepo, *The Book of Awakening: Having the Life You Want by Being Present to the Life You Have.*

provide a template for further deliberate study. Here are a few observations we derived from the interviews.

Marriage and Family

Our interviews found that unconditional love and acceptance from a spouse promoted self-esteem and self-acceptance. Don and Chuck have spouses who say they are happy when their spouses are happy. Chuck said, "Even if I say something [wrong], she understands." And Chuck's wife, Rosemary, agrees. Don's wife, Linda, said, "He consoles me and brings me a glass of wine. This is where we are now." In both cases these couples are the best of friends. Strokes to the left hemisphere that render one with aphasia often don't markedly change a relationship, especially in long-standing, solid marriages.

Don and Chuck had parents they openly loved. They said their parents were caring and generous. Loving parents and loving spouses may be associated with a better outcome and adjustment after a stroke with aphasia. Knowing you are cared for and loved regardless of loss of language skills seemed to bode well for the members of our group.

Humor

Humor is a great help. Peg, Danny's wife, is onto something here. She finds consolation in humor, and she is married to a man whom the group sees as happy-go-lucky. They make a good pair. Peg's insight also applies to the group. When I look around the group, I see that those who laugh heartily and don't take their verbal mistakes so seriously are often the best adjusted. However, at least in our group, they are also the ones who have been living with aphasia longer than those who are more troubled. Two individuals who had their strokes more recently, within two years, seem less happy in their current lives. One individual, at age forty-three, has lost most of his friends since his stroke and says, "F—— them. I haven't seen them, and they have not accounted for themselves." He socializes mostly with his family. He now has a job, which is a godsend and may be an avenue to new friendships. The job certainly has given him a sense of purpose and increased his self-confidence. And now even he can be seen smiling and joking around in group. Perhaps group is a place to lay down your defenses and lighten up a bit.

Sometime I become the butt of a joke in group. Recently we were working on cursive writing. As I instructed the group, I said, "Do not lift your pen from the paper as you write." Chuck challenged me and said, "Then how do you cross a *t* or dot an *i*?" He is always at the ready to make a joke in the group. Chuck, at age eighty-four, also seems to be one of the best-adjusted members.

Upbringing

Some individuals, like Steve and Michael, had very challenging childhoods and then marriages that ended in divorce. In spite of hardships in childhood and marriage, they have warm friendships and strong family relationships. They are both very close to their children and their siblings. They now cope and live well in spite of language difficulties. It may be that they applied what they learned earlier in life to this recent hardship. Whatever helped them overcome previous difficulties continues to help them navigate through this hardship. This aspect of one's character or personality is referred to as resilience in the parlance of developmental psychology and is associated with good outcome.

Find New Meaning

Michael (chapter 4) has committed to helping write a book, this one, with the hope of helping others. "Even one person will make this [project] worthwhile." He has changed his relationships to suit his communication style. He doesn't enjoy large gatherings and instead prefers having lunch with his friends one at a time so he can follow the conversation. He lunches with friends as often as three times a week. He has adapted to what some may see as a loss. But it may be that the relationships he retained are less superficial and more meaningful. He has kept his true friends and shed the rest.

Jason still enjoys larger groups, as long as his wife is there. He laughs. It's fine with him because she enjoys it.

J often says he used to be gregarious, singing and enjoying conversation. He now would rather listen. However, recently he played golf and was paired up with a golfer who also suffered a stroke and had aphasia. This lifted J's spirits; he said it was such a relief to meet someone like himself.

Jana volunteers in her grandchild's classroom. Don enjoys filling his week with university-based therapy and aphasia groups. He is not kidding when he says he's content. Barb has slowed down to smell the roses. She feels more intuitive and peaceful now.

Finding new meaning after a stroke takes time.

Appendix A

Websites on Stroke and Aphasia That May Be Helpful

American Heart Association

http://www.heart.org

Learn more about the American Heart Association's efforts to reduce death caused by heart disease and stroke.

American Speech-Language-Hearing Association

http://www.asha.org

ASHA is the national professional, scientific, and credentialing association for members and affiliates who are speech-language pathologists. You can find information about licensed speech-language pathologists and advice on aphasia.

American Stroke Association

http://www.strokeassociation.org

Learn more about the American Stroke Association and its efforts to reduce death and disability caused by stroke.

Easterseals

http://www.easterseals.com

Easterseals provides exceptional services, education, outreach, and advocacy so people with disabilities can live, learn, work, and play in our communities.

Speech-Therapy Workbooks That Can Be Purchased Online

LinguiSystems

http://www.linguisystems.com/products/product/productmenu
LinguiSystems offers workbooks that address language and apraxia, including *WALC 1-11 Aphasia Rehab Workbook of Activities for Language and Cognition* (https://www.linguisystems.com/products/product/display). These time-tested exercises train the underlying processes of language and cognition with tasks that gradually progress in difficulty.

Language Websites

There are numerous free websites for language and cognitive exercises. Here are a few.

English Page

http://www.englishpage.com
EnglishPage.com offers free English lessons with English grammar and vocabulary exercises online. Hundreds of English lessons to help you learn English.

English Maven

http://www.englishmaven.org
Take free online English lessons and exercises here. English Maven offers hundreds of English grammar and vocabulary lessons to help you study English.

Free Online Aphasia Therapy

http://www.aphasiatherapyonline.com
A free speech-therapy website for aphasia. No sign-up and no cost. Developed by a speech pathologist.

Brain Games

All-Star Puzzles
https://www.allstarpuzzles.com
Over thirty thousand free online puzzles: picture puzzles, Sudoku, quotation puzzles, cryptograms, memory match, and anagram lists.

Lumosity: Brain Games & Brain Training
https://www.lumosity.com
Web-based application that uses games to improve cognitive abilities. Provides information about memory, brain health, and cognition.

BrainHQ
http://www.brainhq.com
Think faster, focus better, and remember more with BrainHQ—clinically proven brain exercises brought to you by Posit Science.

Elevate: Your Personal Brain Trainer
https://www.elevateapp.com
Elevate is a brain-training app designed to improve focus, speaking skills, processing speed, and more. Each person gets a personalized training program.

Communication via the Web with Friends and Family after a Stroke

CaringBridge
https://www.caringbridge.org
The CaringBridge website is a personal health journal for rallying friends and family during any type of health journey.

Alternative and Complementary Therapies

Acupressure: Acupressure (a blend of *acupuncture* and *pressure*) is an alternative-medicine technique derived from acupuncture. In acupressure, physical pressure is applied to acupuncture points by the hand or elbow or with various devices. There are literally hundreds of acupressure points on the body.

Acupuncture: The term *acupuncture* describes a family of procedures involving the stimulation of points on the body using a variety of techniques. The acupuncture technique most often studied scientifically involves penetrating the skin with thin, solid, metallic needles that are manipulated by the hands or by electrical stimulation. Practiced in China and other Asian countries for thousands of years, acupuncture is one of the key components of traditional Chinese medicine.

Essential oils: An essential oil is a concentrated hydrophobic liquid containing volatile aroma compounds from plants. Essential oils are also known as volatile oils, ethereal oils, and aetherolea, or simply as the oil of the plant from which they were extracted, such as oil of clove. An oil is "essential" in the sense that it contains the essence of the plant's fragrance—the characteristic fragrance of the plant from which it is derived.

Massage therapy: This is the manual manipulation of soft body tissues (muscle, connective tissue, tendons, and ligaments) to enhance a person's health and well-being. There are dozens of types of massage-therapy methods (also called modalities).

Restorative yoga: A restorative-yoga sequence typically involves only five or six poses, supported by props such as bolsters, pillows, and blocks that allow you to completely relax and rest. Each pose is held for five minutes or more. Restorative poses include light twists, seated forward folds, and gentle backbends.

Yoga: This is a system of physical postures, breathing techniques, and meditation derived from Hindu spiritual practice but often practiced, especially in Western cultures, to promote bodily or mental control and well-being.

Meditation: This is the act or process of spending time in quiet thought for relaxation or religious purposes. It is the practice of turning your attention to a single point of reference. It can involve focusing on the breath, bodily sensations, or a word or mantra.

Appendix B

GLOSSARY

Acute stroke: A stroke that occurs or develops abruptly. The key feature of an acute stroke is that it starts suddenly and without warning. An acute stroke can be either ischemic or hemorrhagic.

Ankle-foot orthosis (AFO): A short leg brace.

Alzheimer's disease: A type of dementia that causes problems with thinking, memory, and behavior.

Americans with Disabilities Act of 1990 (ADA): US labor law that prohibits unjustified discrimination based on disability. The ADA also requires employers to provide reasonable accommodations to employees who have disabilities and imposes accessibility requirements on public accommodations.

Aneurysm: The stretching of an artery wall into a balloon-like bulge. This may lead to a rupture.

Angiography: A procedure that diagnoses blood clots in the blood vessels. The procedure involves the injection of dye into the groin area. The dye travels up to the brain. Then x-rays photograph the brain's blood vessels.

Anticoagulant: A drug to prevent the blood from clotting. **Warfarin** is an example of this type of drug.

Aphasia: A condition that affects the ability to speak, understand, write, and/or read because of brain damage, including damage caused by a stroke.

Apraxia: A motor speech disorder after a stroke.

Artery: A blood vessel that carries blood away from the heart to other parts of the body.

Atherosclerosis: Also known hardening of the arteries. This is a condition in which scar tissue accumulates in the arteries. The scar tissue can block the blood vessels.

Atherosclerotic plaque: Scar tissue in the arteries.

Atrial fibrillation: Abnormal contractions of the upper chambers of the heart, which leads to ineffective pumping of blood by the heart.

Berry aneurysm: A type of aneurysm that forms in the subarachnoid space underneath the brain, usually at a branch point. When these aneurysms burst, they cause **subarachnoid hemorrhage (SAH)**.

Blood clot: This is the result when the blood tissue begins to collect and harden. When this occurs, it can stop the blood flow and lead to a stroke or heart attack.

Brain stem: This is found at the top of the spinal cord and is responsible for many of the brain functions.

Carotid artery: A large artery in the neck that carries blood to the brain. It is often involved in stroke.

Carotid endarterectomy: A surgical procedure that removes clots that cause blockage in the carotid artery.

Cerebrospinal fluid: Clear fluid that surrounds the brain and the spinal cord inside the spinal column.

Cholesterol: A waxy substance that is found in foods from animal products. It's also manufactured inside the body. (See **low-density lipoprotein [LDL]** and **high-density lipoprotein [HDL]**.)

CT scan (CAT scan): A computerized axial tomography scan. A diagnostic tool that takes images of the inside of the head. CT scan can be valuable in ascertaining whether a stroke is the result of bleeding or blockage.

Dementia: A condition that results in severe memory loss and alters independent functioning.

Diabetes: A condition in which the body is incapable of producing or assimilating insulin. Insulin is needed to produce energy.

Diastolic blood pressure: The lower number of a blood pressure reading. Diastolic blood pressure is a measure taken when the heart relaxes between heartbeats. (See **systolic blood pressure**.)

Electrocardiogram (EKG): A test that measures the health of the heart.

Embolus: A blood clot or other fatty deposit floating in the bloodstream. This material can get stuck, block blood flow, and cause an embolic stroke.

Hemorrhage: Excessive or uncontrolled bleeding from a ruptured blood vessel.

High blood pressure: A condition in which the heart has to work too hard to pump enough blood through the arteries.

High-density lipoprotein (HDL): A fat transporter that carries cholesterol and triglycerides in the body. HDL carries fats to the liver, where they are processed and excreted from the body.

Hypertension: A chronic condition in which the blood pressure flowing through the blood vessels is above the normal range. The normal range is typically 120/80, depending on age. The higher number describes systolic blood pressure, while the lower number measures diastolic blood pressure. Hypertension is the number-one factor causing a stroke. Hypertension is also known as high blood pressure.

Infarction: The obstruction of the blood supply to an organ or region of tissue, typically by a thrombus or embolus, causing local death of the tissue.

Intracerebral: Within the brain.

Intracranial: Within the space inside the skull cavity.

Intracerebral hemorrhage: Bleeding from an artery inside the brain.

Ischemia: Decreased blood flow to an area of the body. Minutes without blood flow to the brain can cause severe brain damage, even death.

Ischemic stroke: A stroke caused by a lack of blood flow, usually because a blood clot has blocked a blood vessel in the brain.

Lipid: Fat found in the blood.

Low-density lipoprotein (LDL): Often called "bad cholesterol," this is one of the fat transporters that carry lipids in the body. It causes atherosclerotic plaque, which can lead to a stroke. Studies show that lower levels of LDL in the blood mean lower risk of stroke.

Magnetic resonance imaging (MRI) scan: MRI scans use magnetic fields and radio waves to produce images. They are used to diagnose certain types of stroke.

Neologism: A neologism is a new word that is coined especially by a person affected with aphasia, is meaningless except to the coiner, and is typically a combination of two existing words or a shortening or distortion of an existing word.

Microaneurysm: An aneurysm that forms in a small artery deep inside the brain.

Neurologist: A doctor who specializes in studying and treating problems with the brain and nervous system.

Occupational therapist: A therapist trained to help individuals who have disabilities due to stroke or other disabilities by teaching them to be independent in their daily activities, whether at home or work.

Physical therapist: A therapist trained to help individuals with disabilities by teaching them to walk again or use a wheelchair and to perform other physical functions.

Plaque: Deposits of fat that build up in the blood vessels and cause damage and blood clots.

Saturated fats: Fats that are typically found in animal products.

Social worker: A health care professional who is trained to help individuals and families cope with their situation and attain helpful resources.

Sodium: A mineral found in many foods. Can cause high blood pressure and stroke.

Spasticity: A condition in which limb muscles contract uncontrollably and painfully.

Speech therapist: A therapist trained to help individuals who have disorders in language processing and/or expression.

Statin drugs: Drugs that simultaneously raise levels of HDL (good cholesterol) and lower levels of LDL (bad cholesterol).

Stroke: A sudden interruption of the blood supply to the brain caused by blockage of a blood vessel or the rupture of a blood vessel.

Subarachnoid hemorrhage (SAH): Bleeding from a ruptured vessel between the skull and the brain.

Subarachnoid space: The narrow space between the skull and the brain. It normally contains cerebrospinal fluid. A subarachnoid hemorrhage is a bleed into this space. The arachnoid is named for its delicate, spider-web-like filaments that extend from its undersurface through the cerebrospinal fluid in the subarachnoid space to the pia mater.

Systolic blood pressure: The higher number in a blood pressure reading. This is a measure of blood pressure when the heart is contracting. (See **diastolic blood pressure**.)

Tissue plasminogen activator (tPA): A clot-dissolving drug approved for the treatment of **ischemic stroke**. This drug should be administered within three hours from the time stroke symptoms began. tPA can cause **intracerebral hemorrhage**.

Transient ischemic attack (TIA): An **ischemic stroke** that doesn't last long enough to cause apparent permanent damage.

Triglyceride: A type of fat in our diet (e.g., in vegetable oil) as well as in our bodies. High triglycerides indicate risk for high blood pressure, high blood sugar, and abnormal cholesterol.

Vascular dementia: A form of dementia caused by a series of small strokes.

Vein: A blood vessel that carries blood to the heart from various parts of the body.

Ventricles of the brain: A communicating network of cavities filled with cerebrospinal fluid (CSF) located within the brain. The ventricular system is composed of two lateral ventricles, the third ventricle, the cerebral aqueduct, and the fourth ventricle.

Warfarin: Drug used to prevent blood clotting.

Glossary Bibliography

Levine, Peter G. *Stronger after Stroke: Your Roadmap to Recovery*, 2nd ed. New York: Demos Health, 2013.

Marler, John R. *Stroke for Dummies*. Hoboken, NJ: Wiley, 2005.

Senelick, Richard C. *Living with Stroke: A Guide for Patients and Families*, 4th ed. Birmingham, AL: HealthSouth Press, 2010.

Appendix C

ADDITIONAL READINGS

Burkman, Kip. *The Stroke Recovery Book: A Guide for Patients and Families.* Omaha, NE: Addicus Books, 2010. This book teaches how the brain works and strokes occur. It explains impairments subsequent to stroke, rehabilitation, and care after stroke for both patients and caregivers. The book has a thorough resource guide.

Byers, Clay. *Will and I.* New York: Farrar, Straus and Giroux, 2016. "I" is the twin of Will, who suffers a catastrophic car accident and then a stroke. This book chronicles the amazing story of his recovery. Notably, he finds a teacher who encourages him to sing to regain his speech.

Doidge, Norman. *The Brain That Changes Itself: Stories of Personal Triumph from the Frontiers of Brain Science.* New York: Viking, 2007. This book focuses on new developments in neuroscience. Neuroplasticity holds great promise for stroke patients, people who have learning disorders, and aging.

Douglas, Kirk. *My Stroke of Luck.* New York: HarperCollins, 2002. This is an easy-to-read story of Kirk Douglas's recovery from stroke. He summarizes his advice in the last chapter, "My Operator's Manual," which includes solid tips such as "Never give up or lose your sense of humor."

Levine, Peter G. *Stronger after Stroke: Your Roadmap to Recovery*, 2nd ed. New York: Demos Health, 2013. This book focuses on stroke recovery, including recovery strategies and the importance of neuroplasticity.

Marler, John R. *Stroke for Dummies*. Hoboken, NJ: Wiley, 2005. This book deals with types of strokes, preventing strokes, treating strokes, and living with a stroke. (At the beginning of the book, the author gives a disclaimer: this book is not about golf!)

McCrum, Robert. *My Year Off*. New York: Broadway Books, Random House, 1998. At forty-two Robert suffered a severe stroke to the right hemisphere of the brain, leaving him with left hemiparesis and an enforced year off alone. This book is for families as well as those who have suffered an "insult to the brain." He asks why and answers that everything has a purpose. He lists dos for the stroke survivor, such as accepting help, trusting yourself, and giving yourself time.

Senelick, Richard C. *Living with Stroke: A Guide for Patients and Families*, 4th ed. Birmingham, AL: HealthSouth Press, 2010. This book addresses risk factors, different types of strokes, recovery, and the family.

Stein, Joel, Julie Silver, and Elizabeth Frates. *Life after Stroke: A Guide to Recovering Your Health and Preventing Another Stroke*. Baltimore: John Hopkins University Press, 2006. The authors use examples from patients to illustrate how stroke occurs and its consequences. They describe both neurological recovery and functional recovery. They include advice on reducing risk factors.

Taylor, Jill Bolte. *My Stroke of Insight: A Brain Scientist's Personal Journal*. New York: Plume, 2006. Taylor, at thirty-seven, suffered a stroke that affected the left hemisphere of her brain. This book documents her eight-year recovery with the help of her mother, who supported her in every way. Along the way, she discovered that relying on the right hemisphere of her brain gave her insight and a new perspective.

Turner, Glenn, with Mark Rosin. *Recognizing and Surviving Heart Attacks and Stroke: Lifesaving Advice You Need Now.* Columbia: University of Missouri Press, 2008. The authors teach the early signs of heart attack and stroke. They describe medical terminology and advice on how to avoid heart attack and strokes. They give thorough education on weight loss, diet, and how to lower cholesterol.

Wanlass, Richard. *Bouncing Back: Skills for Adaption to Injury, Aging, Illness and Pain.* Oxford, United Kingdom: Oxford University Press, 2017. This book is a must-read for anyone adapting to and coping with adjustment after injury, stroke, or aging. It is an easy-to-read guide for step-by-step behavior change.

Zivin, Justin, and John Galbraith Simmons. *tPA for Stroke: The Story of a Controversial Drug.* Oxford, United Kingdom: Oxford University Press, 2011. This book presents a history of tPA (tissue plasminogen activator), a powerful and controversial drug that is the only effective treatment for acute stroke. It chronicles the politics, science, biotech, and development of the drug; the development of protocols; the drug trials; and the advancement to its current use.

Notes

All participants signed release forms to allow publication of their brain scans and the results and interpretations. In some cases, their names have been disguised.

Made in the USA
Columbia, SC
20 November 2017